MAKING A MINDFUL NATION

Making a Mindful Nation

MENTAL HEALTH AND GOVERNANCE
IN THE TWENTY-FIRST CENTURY

JOANNA COOK

PRINCETON UNIVERSITY PRESS

PRINCETON & OXFORD

Published by Princeton University Press
41 William Street, Princeton, New Jersey 08540
99 Banbury Road, Oxford OX2 6JX

press.princeton.edu

All Rights Reserved

ISBN 9780691244471
ISBN (pbk.) 9780691244488
ISBN (e-book) 9780691244495

British Library Cataloging-in-Publication Data is available

Editorial: Fred Appel & James Collier
Production Editorial: Ali Parrington
Jacket/Cover Design: Karl Spurzem
Production: Lauren Reese
Publicity: William Pagdatoon & Charlotte Coyne
Copyeditor: Francis Eaves

Jacket/Cover Credit: Olga Lyubkin / Shutterstock

This book has been composed in Arno

10 9 8 7 6 5 4 3 2 1

CONTENTS

ACKNOWLEDGEMENTS

I COULD NOT HAVE WRITTEN this book without the support and kindnesses of numerous friends, colleagues, students, and institutions.

First and foremost, I am beyond grateful to the mindfulness practitioners who welcomed me into their worlds, personal and professional, and who included me in the ups and downs of their relationships with mindfulness over the years. Their generosity is at the heart of this book.

A British Academy Senior Research Fellowship and a Visiting Fellowship at Stanford University supported the writing of the book, both of which enabled me to develop a first draft. Two of the chapters have appeared elsewhere. Chapter 1 was first published in the *Journal of Global Buddhism* 22 (1) (2021) and material from chapter 5 appears in *Beyond Description* (Heywood and Candea 2023); I am grateful to the editors for their permission to publish the work here.

UCL has provided me with a wonderful home, and I am grateful to my colleagues for their wholeheartedness and passion for anthropology, particularly Allen Abramson, Timothy Carroll, Haidy Geismer, Martin Holbraad, Susanne Keuchler and Charles Stewart. The Medical Anthropology section have been a supportive and exciting group of people with whom to work: Gareth Breen, Joe Calabrese, Sahra Gibbon, Dalia Iskander, David Napier, Aaron Parkhurst, Sara Randall and Carrie Ryan. My brilliant students at UCL have challenged and inspired me throughout the writing of this book, particularly those on the course 'Anthropology of Ethics and Morality', and I am grateful to them for genuinely exciting and exploratory conversations.

A partial list of all those who kindly gave advice and support must include Matei Candea, Nick Evans, Caroline Humphrey, Nick Long, Mathew Thomson and Soumhya Venkatesan. At Stanford, my thanks go to Tanya Luhrmann for unfailing support, encouragement and friendship. And I am very grateful to Leslie Pritchett for providing me with a home, wine and ridiculous amounts of fun during my time in the States. I am humbly obliged to those who read substantial portions of my manuscript and did their best to make them better: Peter Allen, Madeleine Bunting, James Laidlaw and Jon Mair—thanks also to Jon for setting up (and enforcing) pretend chapter deadlines to keep me on track. I thank Fred Appel, James Collier and my two anonymous readers for Press, for believing in this project, and Ali Parrington and Francis Eaves for their careful work on its production.

I am very grateful to my family: to Beatrice, whose birth gave me a hard deadline to work with, my brother, David Cook, for always being there, and to my parents Marcus Cook and Sally Burnley, and their respective partners, Tasha Mundy and Paul Burnley. And to my in-laws, Peter and Jennifer Heywood, and to Bertie the dog. I also give thanks for the extraordinary friendships that have carried me through all of it: with Joanna Beasley, Yasmin Khan, Stefan Moss, Natasha Moscovici, Ella Saltmarshe, Annabelle Stanley, Kary Stewart and Lorna Watson.

Finally, I am indebted most of all to my husband, Paolo Heywood, who has read every draft of every chapter with patience and love, and who is a brilliant thinker, my closest friend, an incredible father and generally the best person with whom to share a life.

MAKING A MINDFUL NATION

If Mindfulness is the Answer, What is the Question?

MINDFULNESS IS EVERYWHERE. Advertisements encourage consumers to 'Breathe in for as long as it takes to read this line. Breathe out for as long as it takes to read this line.' Magazines at supermarket checkouts list meditation in features offering advice on '10 tips for a happier life'. Radio DJs and talk-show hosts interview monks and mindfulness teachers, and books on meditation, psychology and the brain sciences sell in their millions, while tens of thousands of news stories wax lyrical about mindfulness's benefits for stress management in workaday lives (Van Dam et al. 2018, 68). It is now so normal for people to practise mindfulness (or think that they ought to) that if you have an iPhone, you have an inbuilt mindfulness section in your health data app that tells you that 'taking some time to quiet your mind, be in the moment, can make you less stressed and improve your health overall'. In short, learning to 'be present in the moment' is having its moment.

The timing of this meteoric public ascent is noteworthy. Mindfulness is being championed as a prophylactic psychological support at a time of intense public concern about mental health and psychological vulnerability. Depression is the number one cause of disability worldwide (Kousoulis 2019, 2), and the burden of mental health is on the rise (WHO 2020). In the United States, one in four Americans is reported to have a mental or substance use disorder (McCane-Katz 2020) and the National Center for Health Statistics reported a suicide-rate increase of 35 per cent between 1999 and 2018 (Hedegaard, Curtin and Warner 2020). In the UK, it is estimated that up to 10 per cent of the adult population will experience symptoms of depression in any given week and depressive relapse rates are high: following one episode of depression 50 per cent will go on to have a second episode, and 80 per cent of these will go on to have three or more episodes (Singleton et al. 2003). Since 2009 the number of sick days lost to stress, depression and anxiety has increased by 24 per cent and the number lost to serious mental illness has doubled (Mehta, Murphy and Lillford-Wildman 2014). And this rise in mental health challenges is not limited to adult populations. The number of fifteen- to sixteen-year-olds with depression nearly doubled between the 1980s and the 2000s (Nuffield Foundation 2013), and over half of those who experience mental illness in childhood suffer it again as adults (Kim-Cohen et al. 2003; Kessler, Berglund et al. 2005).

Interest in mental health is not limited to clinical conditions. Researchers focusing on positive mental health conceptualise mental health as a spectrum encompassing mental disorder, 'languishing' and 'flourishing' (see Huppert 2009; Keyes 2002a; 2002b; also Huppert 2005);[1] and primary prevention is a central focus of public mental health campaigns that seek to stop mental health problems before they arise. As the Mental Health Foundation states on its website (MHF 2022), '[w]e all have mental health, just as we all have physical health'. Researchers characterise positive mental health, or 'flourishing', as the presence of psychological and social well-being, a categorisation that extends far beyond the absence of mental illness. And they suggest that many of us may be occupying the suboptimal space of 'languishing' most of the time.

By the time I began the fieldwork for this book, a body of research was growing that linked mindfulness to the prevention of mental disorder and the cultivation of positive mental health. Thousands of articles in scientific journals explored the therapeutic potential of mindfulness, examining everything from brain waves to irritability.[2] Evidence was being compiled that suggested that Mindfulness-Based Cognitive Therapy (MBCT) might help large numbers of people experiencing depressive affect and patterns of recurring depression (Baer 2003; Coelho, Canter and Ernst 2007) and three randomised-controlled trials had found that MBCT significantly reduced the risk of depressive relapse (Kuyken et al. 2008; Ma and Teasdale 2004; Teasdale, Segal et al 2000).[3] Clinical studies were investigating the benefits of meditation, motivated by the possibility of reducing stress, increasing productivity, addressing psychological disorders and supporting 'flourishing'. Bolstered by an increasingly healthy evidence base, advocates and practitioners had introduced mindfulness into schools and universities, prisons, the probation service, healthcare institutions and workplaces (public, private and third sector). It is an extraordinary phenomenon that a Buddhist awareness training practice is now being framed as a solution to societal challenges as wide-ranging as criminal recidivism, academic attainment, depressive relapse and workplace absenteeism.

In this book I ask, if mindfulness is the answer, what is the question? What is it that unites the workplace and the prison cell? How are the classroom and the hospital understood, such that they are connected by an awareness practice? And how have mindfulness practitioners come to think of cultivating a kindly relationship with their own minds as a constituent aspect of the 'good life'? How has it happened that mindfulness has become an appropriate support for such a range and variety of different societal challenges? What has changed to lead to this framing? And how have these changes affected how people relate to themselves and to others? To put it another way: if mindfulness is an appropriate practice in every area, from the clinic to the classroom, and for diverse people, from people who are leading healthy, happy lives to those struggling with their mental health in circumstances that are stacked against them, what does this tell us about the questions people are asking about the mind and how they understand themselves in relation to their minds?

Mindfulness provides a window onto a particular moment in which the mind has become a preeminent focus (see McMahan 2008, 201–2). The category of mental health has progressively altered in recent years, shifting from an either/or categorisation of those who do or do not suffer from mental ill-health, to one of an affliction affecting one in four people, to one of a fluctuating condition of all human life. Sometimes described as a shifting landscape, sometimes as a scale, location on which changes, mental ill-health is often now thought of as something that affects all people to a greater or lesser extent at different points in their lives. The expansion of the category of mental health swells the populations for whom it is a concern and transforms responses to address it. 'Mental health' is no longer only relevant for those who would qualify for a mental health diagnosis; in this new categorisation, all people are more or less well at different points in their lives. And emphasis shifts from illness to health: the prevention of illness is met and supported by the active cultivation of positive mental health in order to 'live well'. In this book, I interrogate the consequences of these transformations, examining how people think of themselves, what they think they should do, the values with which mental health is invested, the policies that are created around it and the ways in which the goals of those policies are achieved. Mental health has become a transversal feature of life and one that can be actively supported through dedicated practices. Through my focus on mindfulness, I show how mental health is incorporated into people's relationships with themselves, therapeutic interventions, structures of governance and political campaigns.

An Anthropology of Metacognition

Mindfulness is often thought of as a solitary activity (people sitting still with their eyes shut, perhaps), and is commonly described as an acultural, universal, timeless or ancient practice. But recent anthropological and social scientific work has challenged these assumptions, revealing the historical and cultural processes that inform mindfulness and meditation in diverse contexts. Kirmayer (2015a) has rightly highlighted that adapting techniques like mindfulness from the social contexts in which they originate changes the meaning, nature and effect of their practice; and, as Gajaweera emphasizes (2016) in her work with ethnic and racial minority meditators in Los Angeles, origin traditions do not themselves stay still, and are perpetually subject to proximate and foreign influences. Historians and religious scholars have provided excellent considerations of the development of mindfulness and its relationship to wider religious and secular contexts (see Braun 2022; Husgafvel 2018; McMahan 2008; Nathoo 2019; Wilson 2014; 2017). And anthropologists have demonstrated that mindfulness is informed by normative registers that influence the self-knowledge generated through practice (see Cassaniti 2018; Hedegaard 2020; Mautner 2020; McKay 2019; Myers, Lewis and Dutton 2015; Pagis 2009; 2010; 2019; Vogel 2017; Wheater 2017), providing descriptive accounts of the ways in which interior experiences are socially enabled. Anthropologists have shown, that is, that far from being timeless and universal, mindfulness is fundamentally informed by the cultures and the contexts in which it is ensconced.

Mindfulness, as it is now found in institutions around the world, originated in Buddhist meditation, and the term itself is often taken to be a translation of the Pali word *sati* (see Cassaniti 2018; Gethin 2011 for sustained discussions of this). Beginning in the 1950s in south-east Asia, reformist monks developed, reinvigorated and propagated a form of meditation, *vipassanā*, based on a Buddhist text, *The Mahāsatipatthāna Sutta* (see Braun 2013; Cook 2010a; Jordt 2007). Reformers understood *sati* as an ethically positive perspectival awareness, which could be cultivated through meditative discipline, requiring morality, concentration and wisdom. Therapeutic mindfulness-based interventions are described by their originators as 'marriages' between a conceptual framework from cognitive psychology and quite intensive training in mediation, a 'confluence of two powerful and potentially synergistic epistemologies'

(Williams and Kabat-Zinn 2011, 1). But while the Buddhist roots of mindfulness may be fleetingly referenced in mindfulness courses, mindfulness is most commonly interpreted as a universal human capacity that can be cultivated by practitioners in order to alleviate mental, physical and emotional suffering. Thus, while mindfulness is understood to have originated in Buddhism, it is commonly conceptualised as modern, scientific and secular. And it is framed as a universal and acultural psychological skill that can support the reduction of suffering and the cultivation of mental health.

While there are some disagreements about how mindfulness should be defined (see Mikulas 2011), it is most commonly understood as an awareness-training practice that enables people to '[pay] attention in a particular way, on purpose, in the present moment and non-judgementally' (Segal, Williams and Teasdale 2002, 121). Through daily practice, mindfulness practitioners learn to 'pay attention'; that is, to develop awareness of the patterns of their thoughts, emotions and bodily experiences. This is done 'on purpose' as practitioners intentionally change the focus and style of their attention, by 'non-judgementally' focusing on what they experience in the 'present moment', making emotional experience and the fluctuations of cognition the object of self-conscious reflection without trying to alter that experience. Through this ongoing cultivation of awareness, people intend to relate differently to their experiences and, as a result, to live healthier lives.

Mindfulness gained legitimacy as a secular and therapeutic practice following the development of Mindfulness-Based Stress Reduction (MBSR), an intervention designed by Jon Kabat-Zinn in America in the 1970s to treat chronic disease and pain, though it was only with the development of Mindfulness-Based Cognitive Therapy (MBCT) by Mark Williams, Zindel Segal and John Teasdale in 1991 that mindfulness-based interventions began to influence mental healthcare significantly in the UK (see chapter 1). MBCT is a psychosocial group-based intervention for people who have had three or more depressive episodes but who are currently well. The course is a practice-based training to support participants to identify early signs of depression in order to prevent relapse and to actively maintain their mental health. It encourages participants to develop awareness of small fluctuations in mood, thoughts or bodily experiences, and they learn that developing awareness in this way while they are well has the potential to prevent them relapsing into depression. Practitioners and promotors of mindfulness describe this meta-cognitive ability as a universal human capacity that can be cultivated,[4] and they learn to relate to the mind as a mind, to think about thinking in a peculiarly committed way, by recognising thoughts as 'objects in the mind' and relating to them with kindliness.

Anthropologists have highlighted that attentional and metacognitive skills vary across cultures (see Proust and Fortier 2018) and that how people think about thinking has effects on the strategies that they employ in relation to thought, and on the habits and skills that they seek to cultivate in order to influence the direction or quality of their attention (see Cassaniti and Luhrmann 2014; Hirschkind 2001; 2006; Luhrmann 2012, xxi; Mair 2018). They have shown that people have clear ideas about the nature of thought and how they ought to relate to it, and that these ideas are embedded in particular relationships and practices. Anthropological accounts reveal the effortful practice that people make to attend to attention in particular ways; that people wilfully and actively cultivate attentional skills in order to effect change in their lives. The pan-human capacity for metacognition is invested with specific cultural and attitudinal values through the practice of mindfulness. And it is the particular way in which people relate to their minds (and not just the fact that they do so) that is central to mindfulness. The mindfulness practitioners who are the focus of this book intentionally cultivate forms of awareness and attentional focus through mindfulness training. They learn that they *can* have a relationship with their own minds, and they learn techniques for developing a particular form of effortful attention to the mind that involve repetitive practice, requiring ongoing training in metacognitive awareness. They think that cultivating metacognitive ability, or learning to 'make friends' with one's own mind through self-reflective practice, is of benefit to all people in the maintenance of mental health, whether or not they have ever received a mental health diagnosis. For them, living well is characterised by metacognitive skill, attentional training and the cultivation of a kindly relationship with one's own objectified mind. In chapters 2 and 3 I delineate the particular attitudinal dispositions that characterise the metacognitive skill that mindfulness practitioners cultivate. In mindfulness as a therapeutic intervention and as a daily practice, the attitudinal quality of kindliness imbues metacognitive ability and is central to the objectification of the mind.

Psychological Governance and the Ethical Turn

In the 1950s, depression was so rare that pharmaceutical companies saw no benefit in investing money in its treatment (Healy 1997). And yet, by the 1990s, the second most prescribed drug in the United States was the antidepressant

Prozac (Elliott 2018). While statistics about the projected costs, prevalence and severity of depression all point to an emerging public health crisis and provide grounds for immediate action, such as funding, research and intervention to support individuals and communities, anthropologists have argued that cause and effect work the other way: that depression is 'socially constructed' through changes to diagnostic criteria, increased awareness, and the medicalisation and commercialisation of mental states (see Hirschbein 2014; Kitanaka 2011). Social scientists have characterised shifting dynamics of mental health classification and presentation as a diagnostic (rather than a psychological or biological) epidemic, finding in escalating mental health statistics a 'contagion of representation' (Mattingly 2017; see also Grinker 2007). Such social constructionist accounts provide illuminating insights into the cultural and historical conditions that inform the way that categories of representation such as 'mental health', 'depression' or 'anxiety', are constructed, charting the new forms of biosociality established around changes in diagnostic criteria as scientific research is targeted, rights and services are expanded and people come together in activist movements and self-help groups organised around a particular illness or disability (Rabinow 1996; Rose and Rabinow 2006).

Important studies of the cultural history of psychology have highlighted how truth discourses about human character are taken up by different authorities, informing strategies for intervention and the ways in which individuals work on themselves in support of individual or collective health (see Cushman 1995; Danziger 1990; Rose 1985; 1996b). Psychological terms, diagnoses, explanations, values and judgements thus get entangled with a more general contemporary 'regime of the self' as the prudent yet enterprising individual actively shapes his or her life course through acts of choice (see Novas and Rose 2000). As psychological thinking expands, it informs the habits, values and obligations of the self-sufficient, 'responsibilised' citizen who is able to withstand the uncertainties of modern life (Brown 2003; Cruikshank 1996; Rose 1996a, 1996b). In such a reading, it is people's *freedom* that enables them to become objects of governance, because it binds them 'to a subjection that is more profound because it *appears* to emanate from our autonomous quest for ourselves, it *appears* as a matter of freedom' (Rose 1990, 256, emphasis added). The intensified attention to the inner life of psychological subjectivity is, as Rose revealed in his seminal work, intimately connected to the marriage between political agendas and 'the personal projects of individuals to live a good life' (ibid., 10; see also Kleinman et al. 2011). Such approaches afford us the opportunity to examine one form of relationship between self-governance and social forces: the influence of psychological knowledge and technologies for the identification and management of populations, and the influence of expert knowledge in the creation of psychological subjectivity. Psychological knowledge doesn't just describe experience; it also creates and shapes subjects, informing what people think they know about themselves and what it is to be human; and this influences the ways in which they relate to themselves and others.

Where I differ from such approaches is in placing the emphasis of my analysis on first-person experiences of mental health in order to reflect on the categories and structures of governance to which they are constitutively related. In what follows I show that the micro-level efforts that people make to support their mental health, to engage in intentional projects of cognitive and emotional discipline in order to prevent mental ill-health and to promote psychological well-being and flourishing are intimately related to macro-level projects of governance and social structure. Transformations in social services, institutional structures and governmental agendas reflect and contribute to the everyday efforts that people make to attend to their psychological selves. In what follows, I examine how transformations in the category of mental health are central to the reimagining of psychological subjects, the reshaping of techniques of governance and the refashioning of the relationship between parliamentarians and citizen-subjects. And yet, I am in no way arguing that people are *determined* by the social or material forces in which they are ensconced. In fact, this book may be read as a critique of the 'neoliberalism made 'em do it' arguments that circulate around psychological subjectivity and self-governance. Rather, I examine the social processes by which mental health is lived, the normative values that inform it and the practices of self-cultivation by which it is addressed. That is, I extend my analysis beyond the Althusserian 'interpellation' of changing social categories and expert practices to examine the values and efforts with which people navigate the world, and the ethical complexity and cultural particularity of so doing (see also Cook 2023). For example, in the transformations in the category of depression from an acute to a relapsing or recurring condition, or the shift in the category of mental health from relevant for certain at-risk populations to a constituent aspect of life for everyone, how do people's relationships with themselves and others change, what values inform their efforts to live well, and what is the lived experience of these?

In this approach, this book takes inspiration from the recent ethical turn in anthropology (Faubion 2001a; Laidlaw 2002; Lambek 2000a). The development of the anthropology of ethics is seen by some as a move away from earlier culturalist claims that people think or behave in certain ways because of the society, culture or ideology in which they find themselves (Heywood 2017; Laidlaw 2002).[5] A foundational claim of the anthropology of ethics is not that ethics or morality have a universal content or are constituted by any particular configuration of values. Rather, it claims that people are evaluative: that they hold themselves to different understandings about what is right and wrong, and that they reflect and deliberate on these things (Laidlaw 2014, 3). People exercise this reflective capacity in their considerations about best courses of action, their choices between possible goods, and as a way of accounting for risk, responsibility and consequences. They think about how they ought to live, and this deliberation influences the ways in which they relate to themselves, the practices they undertake, their interactions with others and the choices that they make.

Drawing inspiration from this, I consider psychological subjectivity from the perspective of its 'potentialities as well as its repressive normativities' (Mattingly 2014b, 203). I ask, 'Are there ways of interrogating the moral universalisms of modernity, or technologies of governance, without completely discounting optimism, self-reflection and aspiration?' That is, as Mattingly puts it (2014b, 203),

> Without a strong theory of the human subject as a complex moral agent capable of *acting upon history* (even within a history that also makes her) as well as an agent compelled to *respond* to history, including the small histories that comprise ordinary life, then we, as scholars, miss a great deal about how social life takes shape, what morally matters to people, and even how social change might occur.

My starting point, therefore, is not to take the will of the individual and her capacity to reflect on how she might wish to live and work towards that aim as symptoms of broader knowledge practices or social forces. Instead, I examine the ways in which people negotiate their lives and the ethical potential of the worlds in which they find themselves. That is, I propose that efforts to realise the good life in how people relate to themselves may be explored from the ground up, as well as the top down. Transformations in mental health, the obligations that these entail and the possibilities that they offer involve not only changes in categories, but changes in values, norms and ethical practices. In taking this approach, I seek to account for those aspects of self-cultivation practices and engagement with psychological knowledge that lie beyond formal institutional structures and are motivated by optimistic, hopeful or even utopian ideas about the human condition. And I examine the ways in which people might work to bring something new into being, as much in their relationships with themselves as in political campaigns, and the reasons they might have for so doing.

The Ethics and Instrumentalism of Mental Health

As I have pointed out above, the popularity of mindfulness is bolstered by an increasing evidence base that suggests that mindfulness-based interventions are effective in a range of areas. It is fair to say that, without randomised controlled trials and advanced statistical analyses reporting the 'efficacy' of meditation practice, mindfulness-based initiatives would not have received endorsement from the National Institute for Health and Care Excellence (NICE), would not have been mandated on the UK National Health Service (NHS) and would not be being discussed in the UK parliament as an appropriate response to policy challenges in civil society. But this pragmatic and instrumentalist framing of mindfulness is only part of the picture. At the same time as mindfulness is being witnessed as a targeted intervention for specific populations, it is also being described as a practice for living well, flourishing and 'waking up' to life that is appropriate for everyone. Awareness and attention characterise both the prognosis of and the cure for the challenges of modernity (see Cook 2018; Pedersen, Albris and Seaver 2021): stressed-out lives are hampered by the unhealthy encounter between innate cognitive weakness and radical transformations in the structure of social life, leading to anxiety, emotional numbness and the reactivity of cognitive bias. 'Coming to our senses' through mindfulness, as Jon Kabat-Zinn's celebrated book (2005) is titled, means reconnecting with immediate phenomena, reinhabiting one's direct experiences by cultivating awareness of bodily sensations. One is supposed to cook mindfully, wash the dishes mindfully or wait for the bus mindfully. This emphasis on mindful awareness in daily life far exceeds the short-term management of illness. Rather, the prevention of illness and the promotion of health rest on a fundamental shift in the relationship that a practitioner has with herself and her routine experiences.

As people engage with practices like mindfulness, they invest them with their own values, shaping the taken-for-granted nature of ongoing transformations in the category of mental health. For the people discussed in this book, mindfulness is not transcendent, but ameliorative, a 'this-worldly' means for living well that they think of as both pragmatic and ethical: a means for improving capacities and a capacity in its own right. They think that mindfulness extends from formal practices into daily life and that a mindful relationship with oneself is informed by virtuous dispositions of friendliness, patience and compassion. They also think that, properly supported by evidence, costed and communicated, mindfulness has the potential to help large numbers of people. In a mental health landscape increasingly characterised by an emphasis on preventative healthcare, cultivating a healthy relationship with one's own mind is described as both an evidence-based 'technique' and an ethical practice: Mindfulness is simultaneously promoted as a pragmatic and targeted intervention to address the high levels of stress and anxiety found in diverse populations and it is engaged with as a way to 'wake up' to life.

The coexistence of these two languages, of utility and ethics, seems counterintuitive: one represents the 'bottom line' of a highly rationalised, impersonal and measurable modern world. The other points to subjective experience and inner orientation, often promoted as a supportive response to the alienation and disenchantment resulting from the harshness of that same modernity (see Nolan 1998, 285). I argue that, in the logic of preventative healthcare, instrumental questions about 'fixing' are blended with Socratic questions about the good life. In combining the psychological/medical question, 'How can mental ill-health be prevented/alleviated?' and the ethical questions, 'How can I live well?' and 'What is flourishing?', instrumental concerns about alleviation of suffering and deliberation about the good life are merged. Mental health is simultaneously framed as an epidemic that requires action and as 'something we all have', and mindfulness is engaged with as both a preventative intervention for those most at risk of mental ill-health and as a practice that enables people to live more 'fully', one that is as personally relevant for cognitive psychologists as it is for patients. In such a reframing of mental health, it is unsurprising that people in diverse areas of life take up mindfulness to address seemingly different challenges, as questions particular to a given issue (criminal recidivism, worker presenteeism, etc.) become interwoven with ethical questions about the 'good life'.

Combined, the logics of these developments have had a profound impact on the ways in which mental health is understood and addressed. It is no longer something that can be 'fixed': we all have mental health, all of the time; it is not a disease that can be removed, but rather, something to be tended to and maintained in order to prevent a slide into mental ill-health and to support a flourishing and happy life. Two correlated effects result from this shift. First, not all mental health is to be treated medically. While acute depressive episodes can be treated with antidepressant medication, an emphasis on the cultivation of positive mental health is not limited to a strictly medical domain. Most therapeutic work escapes the domain of psychiatrists, even though they may endorse it or undertake some of it themselves. And second, the category of mental health is expanded to encompass both the suffering of mental illness and the ups and downs experienced by all people in daily life. We all now have mental health, and we can all do things actively to support it. This expansion of the category of mental health makes it a transversal issue, affecting patients, psychologists and politicians alike, as preventative supports for positive mental health neutralise or sidestep the antimonies of medicalisation: between health and illness, between normal life and pathology, between living well and preventing symptoms and between ethical practice and instrumentalism.

The interaction between incommensurate ethical and economic values extends from personal practices of self-cultivation into contemporary governmental interest in mental health much more broadly. In the second half of this book, I focus on two recent changes in policy development in the UK that exemplify this. First, in an era of evidence-based policy-making, political deliberation increasingly draws on academic research in its commitment to 'what works'. Governmental policy on mental health is informed by evidence from the psychological, social and economic sciences as policy makers seek to develop costed, evidence-based and effective policies. Second, in response to charges of technocratic governance, evidence-based policy deliberation occurs through structures of participatory governance, based on the orchestration of governmental, third sector, academic, lay and professional collaboration. The recategorisation of mental health as a transversal concern informs this emphasis on evidence-based participatory governance: Civil servants and politicians understand themselves to be as vulnerable to mental health issues as other citizens and the evidence from the psychological sciences is deliberated in participatory fora as transversally relevant. The rationalism of evidence-based psychological services for the prevention and treatment of illness and the Romanticism of the potential of self-work for living more fully coalesce in the expanded category of mental health as a transversal issue, and in the popularity of mindfulness as an evidence-based ethical practice. Mindfulness is *both* an instrumentalised intervention *and* an ethical practice; a pragmatic support for mental health and a 'way of being' that infuses everyday life. Furthermore, as

I will show, it is important to the people discussed in this book that mindfulness maintains this multiplicity of values as this 'both/and' characterisation of mindfulness extends from personal practice into policy discussion and political deliberation.

Researching Cultures of Mindfulness

I first encountered mindfulness while I was finishing my book on Buddhist meditation (Cook 2010a). I had spent years researching how monks and nuns in a monastery in northern Thailand cultivate insight into the Buddhist truths of impermanence, suffering and non-self. Through intensive meditation practice, monastics intentionally cut attachment to a delusional sense of self, and progress towards enlightenment. Writing the book had been a labour of love over a number of years, during which time I participated in a regular meditation group in Cambridge, UK. Once a week, six or seven of us would meet to meditate, listen to a *dhamma* talk and eat cake. It was here that I first heard about MBCT, and I was struck by the fact that this therapeutic intervention shared direct links with the soteriological discipline of the Thai monastery (see chapter 1). While the ink was drying on my book about Thai renunciation and meditative discipline, people across the UK were engaging with meditation as a scientifically verifiable support for living well in a stressful world. And the meditative practices that were central to ascetic discipline and enlightenment in the monastery were being used by my companions to support their mental health and to navigate the daily ups and downs of romantic relationships, work stresses and family responsibilities.

As in America, in Britain mindfulness was the focus of scientific research and media interest at the time. But while mindfulness grew in popularity in the US over the same period (see Wilson 2014; 2017), it is possible to make a case for Britain as the epitome of the 'mindful nation'. Unlike in the US, mindfulness in Britain receives public funding, and its uptake has been facilitated by centralised deployment through the NHS and the country's relatively smaller size. Mindfulness-Based Cognitive Therapy (MBCT) is available on the NHS as a preventative intervention for recurrent depression and is now taught as a master's degree for healthcare professionals at British universities. In 2013 mindfulness courses were established in Westminster for parliamentarians and parliamentary staff and, at the time of writing, over 250 parliamentarians and 450 staff have completed an eight-week course. In 2014, parliamentarians and advocates set up an All-Party Parliamentary Group (APPG) in Westminster to investigate the policy potential for mindfulness in the criminal justice system, education, healthcare and the workplace.

The fieldwork upon which this book is based spanned each of these sites: mindfulness courses for people suffering from recurrent depression and anxiety; postgraduate courses for mindfulness-based therapists; parliamentarians' mindfulness practice; and political advocacy for mindfulness in public policy. In 2013 I began participant observation with two cohorts on a two-year mindfulness therapist training programme at a university in the UK. Over the course of three years, fieldwork involved engaging with the full pedagogy of the programme as I sought to embed myself in training: personal practice, participation in the eight-week MBCT course, regular practice periods, silent retreats, guided reading, lectures and workshops, peer presentations, tutorials, supervised practice, reflective diaries, essays, peer observation and out-of-school activities. The two cohorts of students with whom I worked were made up of healthcare professionals from a range of different backgrounds, including therapists, nurses, GPs (general practitioners), carers and psychologists. They were enthusiastic and excited about my research. With their consent, I sought to understand the struggles that they faced in training, and subsequently in practice, and to make sense of the ways in which mindfulness informed their personal and professional practice over the course of years (see Cook 2017; 2020). During this time I also conducted participant observation on eight-week MBCT courses with people who had been referred by healthcare professionals, usually to address issues of recurrent depression and anxiety. In the UK, people who wish to participate in an MBCT course on the NHS must be referred via the Depression and Anxiety services, their GP or local Mental Health Assessment Teams (see Cook 2015). In order to research it as a structured learning process for both therapists and participants, experiential knowledge of mindfulness was of paramount importance, and fieldwork involved a methodological commitment to practice-based research, a focus that shares interesting parallels with the place of practice in mindfulness-based interventions themselves (see Cook 2020).

The other focus of my research was the British parliament. From May 2014 I worked with the group of parliamentarians and volunteer advocates who established the Mindfulness All-Party Parliamentary Group (APPG), beginning an eighteen-month inquiry into the benefits of mindfulness in the areas of health, education, criminal justice and the workplace (see Cook 2016). Following this period, volunteer advocates drafted a report, *Mindful Nation UK*, gathering evidence for mindfulness-based interventions across diverse sectors of civil society in the UK. Over the course of the fieldwork I made dozens of trips to Westminster either to meet advocates and parliamentarians or to attend the meetings and events to which I had been invited, and much of the work in parliament was organised around scheduled meetings and interviews. Each time, the 'imponderabilia' of life—the catch-up in the café before a meeting, the conversation in the halls afterwards—provided important insights into people's engagement with mindfulness. But Westminster is not a place where one can just 'show up' and 'hang out'; one needs a good reason to be there. Entering through the Cromwell Green entrance on the other side of the building from the river Thames, visitors are asked by a police officer or a visitor assistant what they are there for or whom they are there to meet before being allowed to move through security. On busy days, this can take up to an hour, and requires patience. Each person is given a visitor security pass before putting all bags and coats through the airport-style X-ray machines and stepping through a metal detector. Once on the other side of security, one comes to Westminster Hall, the oldest building on the parliamentary estate. Here, one sees the business of Westminster unfolding—tours of schoolchildren being shown around, groups of constituents waiting for meetings, businessmen and military personnel, interns and politicians, all under a magnificent hammer-beam roof and on flagstones literally marked by the events of history. Strikingly, and importantly for my argument in this book, the practice-based fieldwork methods that were central to my work with therapists and MBCT participants were vital for fieldwork in Westminster as well, and one of the most unanticipated experiences of fieldwork was meditating in Westminster Palace with MPs (members of the House of Commons), peers (members of the House of Lords) and special advisors. Every meeting of the APPG was prefaced with a mindfulness practice, as advocates, parliamentarians and parliamentary staff joined invited experts and stakeholders in mindfulness practice, their doing so informed by their ongoing personal practice.

The most intensive periods of fieldwork were the three years on the therapist training programme when I was participating in training and retreats, the period of the inquiry process in parliament when I was attending hearings and the subsequent work with advocates as they drafted the *Mindful Nation* report. During this period, from 2013 to 2015, I spent part of each week with participants on courses, therapists in training, advocates and parliamentarians. On most occasions, I joined the people I was working with in meditation. I had had significant experience of various meditative practices prior to beginning this research, and my earlier work on Thai monasticism had involved ongoing practice in intensive Burmese *vipassanā* (insight) (see Cook 2010a, 19; 2010b). But while mindfulness in Britain shares historical roots with the meditative discipline of the Thai monastery where I worked (see chapter 1), I was surprised by how far the two differed. Whereas in the monastery, meditation was characterised by renunciation through meditative discipline, mindfulness in this research was focused on kindliness towards oneself and, over the course of fieldwork, this emphasis on 'softening' profoundly influenced my personal practice. My own meditative experience is not the focus of this book, but it was a key part of my methodology and I spent hundreds of hours meditating with research participants in each of the field sites.

Over the course of the research, I conducted seventy-three recorded interviews, collected formal and informal histories and attended regular and ad hoc meetings. While employing formal research methods in each of the four areas (mindfulness courses, therapist training, appointments in Westminster and advocacy meetings) was important, such methods are, by and large, in addition the anthropologist's methodological bread-and-butter: participant observation. The less accountable activity of myriad 'small moments' was vital for the research. These included 'hanging out' on lunch breaks, dinners, social events, picnics, walks by the river, sober raves, sitting together waiting for a meeting to begin or debriefing afterwards. This anthropological hanging out involved both the formal research methods of life histories and interviews, and participation in shared practices such as meditation training, group therapy or (countless) meetings. But it also involved innumerable 'small moments', noting what comes up in the in-between spaces, when I was meeting others not to conduct an interview, but simply to spend time together.

Through long-term ethnographic research, I sought to understand how the people with whom I work engage with mindfulness. I have pseudonymised everyone who appears in this book, except for those cases in which their statements are a matter of public record. Most of the relationships that inform what follows were intimate and ongoing, and I have attempted to represent the values and practices of the people with whom I work as faithfully as I am able to. For many of the people featured in this book, mindfulness is a practical activity, a way of becoming familiar and friendly with the patterns of the mind, and emotional and somatic responses. They engage with mindfulness as a support for their mental health and as a way of cultivating a skilful engagement with life, and they believe that they are healthier and happier as a result of their practice. They think that mindfulness reduces psychological suffering and changes the relationship they have with themselves, and they are committed to practising mindfulness themselves, to teaching other people to practise it and to promoting it in society. Practitioners across society promote mindfulness, from the grass-roots to the government, as both a targeted and pragmatic antidote to the more terrible effects of anxiety and depression and as a form of awareness training associated with well-being and flourishing, broadly conceived.

In chapter 1 I develop a history of mindfulness in the UK, tracing contemporary framings of mindfulness through the ongoing dialogue between Buddhism and psychology over the last century and a half. I show that contemporary mindfulness developed as a scientifically verifiable method for living more 'fully', steeped in the tensions between rationalist calls for empirical certainty and Romantic calls for meaning and experience, and I argue that the threads of Romanticism and rationalism are woven through preventative mental healthcare more broadly. In chapter 2 I examine the recent reframing of depression from being an acute to a relapsing or recurring condition, and the development of Mindfulness-Based Cognitive Therapy (MBCT), a long-term psychosocial intervention for those most vulnerable to relapse. Focusing on the structured learning process of the eight-week MBCT course, I examine how participants learn to relate differently to their experience and to depression. Participants learn that there is a cognitive component to depressive relapse, they cultivate reflexive awareness of their own thoughts, feelings and bodily sensations, and they work to develop a relationship with themselves and their experiences that is kind.

The emphasis on preventative mental healthcare in MBCT reflects broader changes in the category of mental health in Britain, as concern about mental health extends beyond the purview of therapy into the activities of daily life. In chapter 3 I focus on the ways in which mindfulness-based therapists integrate mindfulness into their daily lives simultaneously to prevent mental ill-health, to navigate the ups and downs of life and, as they say, to 'live fully'. Mindfulness practitioners learn metacognitive theories and strategies (what people think about thinking, and what they think they should do about it), and these inform their efforts to cultivate habits of awareness that will transform the ways in which they experience ordinary life. I extend this argument in chapter 4, focusing on the development of mindfulness classes for parliamentarians in the British parliament and the influence of popular psychology books. I show that politicians, peers and government advisors recognise their own experiences of stress, depression and anxiety in popular psychological representations of mental health. Through their mindfulness practice, parliamentarians seek to live well in a highly stressful professional world by cultivating a metacognitive relationship with their own experience.

In chapter 5, I argue that the transversal relevance of mental health links practices of psychological self-cultivation, such as mindfulness, with macro-level state agendas and governmental techniques. Focusing on the Mindfulness APPG, I interrogate the wider governmental trends of evidence-based policy-making and participatory governance, showing that, in the APPG, experts and parliamentarians took on a participant's as well as an observer's point of view as they related mindfulness and mental health to themselves and their own actions. Throughout, mindfulness was presented as simultaneously rational and ethical, as an evidence-based intervention that 'works', and a personally transformative practice. The APPG inquiry process culminated in the launch of the *Mindful Nation* report. In chapter 6, I focus on the drafting of *Mindful Nation* by a group of volunteer advocates who had no previous experience of political advocacy. I examine the relationship between the ethical value that mindfulness held for volunteers and the economic values that underpinned the governmental technologies with which they engaged, and I argue that the political case for mindfulness was produced through the ongoing relationship between personal ethics, normative imperatives and new technologies of governance, in a non-linear process informed by ethical, epistemological and economic agendas.

Making a Mindful Nation is an ethnographic study of what happens when mental health becomes a site for self-conscious work. I argue that the popularity of mindfulness is, in part, a result of broader transformations in ideas about the self, mental health and human flourishing. In the UK, people across society have increasingly come to think of mental health as 'something we all have' and something that can be actively supported through cultivating a kindly relationship with their own minds: they think that they can effect positive change on themselves, their habits, their impulses and their reactions by learning to relate differently to their minds. It is a culturally new phenomenon to think of the cultivation of attention and awareness, learning to develop a metacognitive relationship with one's own mind, as a central constituent of the good life. I demonstrate that mental health has become a transversal issue, impacting politicians as much as the populations that they serve: learning to relate to the mind in a kindly way is thought to be of benefit to all people in the maintenance of mental health, whether or not they have ever received a mental health diagnosis. I show that the ways in which people represent mental health, the distinctions that they make, and the solutions that those distinctions lead to, have changed; and I examine how the logics of preventative mental healthcare are incorporated into people's relationships with themselves, therapeutic interventions, structures of governance and political campaigns. The popularity of mindfulness is testimony to its relationship to these larger transformations in the category of mental health, including a remarkable upswing in public and political interest in the mind as an object of governance, by both the self and others.

1

A Genealogy of the 'Present Moment'

ON A TUESDAY evening in October 2015, the parliamentary report *Mindful Nation UK* was launched in Westminster. Mindfulness advocates, civil servants, parliamentarians, journalists and professionals from across the public and private sectors packed into the Attlee Room in Portcullis House for the event, closing their eyes for a guided meditation practice before listening to invited talks from clinical psychologists, schoolchildren and parliamentarians. Mindfulness, an awareness training practice originating in Buddhism, was the focus of intense public and political interest at the time. As the press release for the event put it, 'the nation is facing a mental health crisis', and preventative strategies such as mindfulness 'have a crucial role to play in reducing the burden of mental ill-health on individual wellbeing and the economy'. The secretary of state for education, Nicky Morgan, told the audience that young people are under increased pressures as a result of online life: 'we can't uninvent technology [...] but we can give our young people the resilience, the persistence, the grit, the determination, the self-esteem and the confidence to make sure they can tackle the challenges of the twenty-first century'. She was followed by the health minister, Alistair Burt, who echoed the need for a policy focus on mental health:

> It is vital we do all we can to improve mental health. [...] Mindfulness plays a big part in this, particularly in preventing mental health problems early on, and helping to prevent relapses. [...] Young people need ways to build resilience and recognise the early signs of mental ill-health.

Ministers' commitment to prophylactic psychological support speaks to broader concerns about mental health and psychological vulnerability in the

UK and abroad (see Cook 2018). Mindfulness, for both government ministers, sat squarely within what they identified as a need for interventions that prevent mental health problems from developing and that encourage forms of psychological resilience.

Beginning around the mid-2000s, mindfulness meditation began to appear in popular media in Britain and America on a regular basis (see Conclusion). Journalists were reflecting a growing interest in the potential for meditation to support people in diverse walks of life. Mindfulness was being introduced into non-religious institutions, such as schools, hospitals and prisons, and people were picking up on it on their own, facilitated by the development of popular apps, private courses, local drop-in sessions and a growing literary genre of guided self-practice. In Britain, mindfulness was being interpreted as a positive intervention for societal problems as wide-ranging as depressive relapse, criminal recidivism, children's academic performance and worker burn-out, in part because of the promise it offered to forms of psychological resilience, a broad aspiration that informs much contemporary debate about preventative healthcare.

In the *Mindful Nation* report, mindfulness is presented as one way of 'supporting wellbeing and resilience across the population as a prevention strategy to keep people well' (MAPPG 2015a, 19). It is believed to help those who practise it cope with life (from stress, anxiety and depression to impulse control, emotional regulation and intellectual flexibility). Mindfulness is understood to be a scientifically verified way of cultivating a skilful engagement with life, configured as a technique of self-cultivation to support mental health. Practising mindfulness is associated in the UK with an aspiration towards living a life in which one is fully 'present'. Bringing awareness to the present moment, learning to 'be' with what is, without trying to fix or change anything, is described often as bringing a 'freshness' to lived experience, a direct perception of the world. In the context of preventative healthcare, this ability to relate differently to life events is associated with psychological resilience (see chapter 6).

How has it come about that an awareness training practice originating in Buddhism is being undertaken in parliament and is the focus of policy discussion on psychological resilience in Britain? And, given the unprecedented popularity of mindfulness beyond Westminster, how have British people come to think of cultivating a kindly relationship with their own minds as a valuable endeavour? In this chapter, I take a genealogical approach to the 'present moment', examining the historical development of truth claims about the nature of Buddhism and psychology in Britain since the nineteenth century. I use 'genealogy' in the Foucauldian sense of exploring those things that 'we tend to feel [are] without history' (Foucault 1994, 369). Rather than narrate the progressive development of knowledge about psychological resilience, I point to the complex and interwoven connections that led us to the idea that paying attention to the present moment is psychologically beneficial.[1] In so doing, I uncover the contingency of what might appear to be necessity, and the unexpected linkages by which truth claims about Buddhism and psychology are produced. I reveal some of the shifting ways in which Buddhism, meditation and psychology have been imagined in Britain in order to account for changing understandings of mental health and mindfulness, and their central focus in media, political and popular discourse today.

I hope to demonstrate that contemporary understandings of mindfulness as a universal tool for psychological resilience are informed by a long cultural history. Beginning my narrative in the nineteenth century, I unpack how meditation came to be understood as 'the heart of Buddhism' in Britain and in Europe more widely, and the development of mindfulness as a scientifically verifiable psychological means to live life 'more fully'. From the nineteenth century, scholarly treatises and popular accounts characterised Buddhism as undoubtedly exotic but also surprisingly modern, and resonant with the conditions of uncertainty and transformation that characterised Europe at the time (Masuzawa 2005, 121). I show that Victorian interest in moral rationality led to interpretations of Buddhism as a science-compatible and ethicised religion, but that this was matched too by the nineteenth-century fascination with the occult, spiritual experience and magic. Buddhism was simultaneously understood as compatible with science and informed by Romantic principles of 'present-centeredness'. Psychological interpretations of meditation were influenced by two constituents of Romantic thought: a deep concern that modernity is leading to isolation, atomisation and ill-health; and an emphasis on a quality of engagement with 'ordinary' experience to transcend the ills of modernity.[2] Practising meditation came to be explicitly associated with an aspiration towards living a life in which one is fully 'present'. The seemingly antithetical cultural and intellectual trends of rationalism and Romanticism both thus conditioned orientalist engagement with and understanding of Buddhism, psychology and meditation practice.

Tracing the geometry of these trends and the ways in which they have informed the remarkable uptake of mindfulness in contemporary Britain sheds light on current concerns about mental health and psychological resilience. In response to the seemingly intractable and complex policy problems of mental health, political interest in 'resilience' focuses on capabilities and practices of awareness in preventative interventions. As Chandler writes in his description of resilience-thinking (2014, 4), 'in a rapidly changing world, success is not based so much upon a store of acquired knowledge but upon the capacities of self-reflection and reflexive understanding of how one needs to adapt in an ever-shifting environment'. Psychologically resilient subjects are encouraged to relate differently to limitation through practices of self-governance in a non-linear, complex landscape. Thus, I propose that a choice between rationalism and Romanticism in contemporary debates about mindfulness and mental health might be a false one (see also Albanese 2007; Foucault 1984): calls for rationalism in one direction and re-enchantment in another may be taken as coeval and dominant trends in contemporary life. I unpack this by examining the ways in which currents of empiricism and enchantment have informed the ongoing dialogue between Buddhism and psychology in Britain over the last century and a half.

Enlightenment Values and Romanticism

During the nineteenth century British philologists began to interpret Buddhism as largely compatible with the basic tenets of the European Enlightenment (see Snodgrass 2009). Philological work on Buddhism at the start of the nineteenth century uncovered a 'pure' or 'original' Buddhism as a trans-local universalist textual world religion, detached from cultural context, and the person of the Buddha as a humanist, non-sectarian and rational historical founder. Almond sums this up neatly when he says that for scholars of the time, 'the Buddha was an ideal Victorian gentleman' (Almond 1988, 77–78, 79; see also Snodgrass 2009). Various strands of religious practice in central, south, south-east and east Asia came to be identified as part of a religion that was comparable with the Abrahamic 'world religions' of Islam, Judaism and Christianity. Buddhism met the criterion of having a founding figure in the legendary but historical Prince Gautama, and possessed an impressive body of scriptural writings in ancient Asian languages written after Gautama's death. European scholars began to identify genealogical relations between varied and seemingly discrete traditions across the breadth of Asia, from Ceylon, Burma, Siam, Japan, China and Tartary (Almond 1988). Buddhism was interpreted as an ethical religion which emphasised rational self-perfection and compassion towards others, thereby reflecting the values and desires of Victorian scholars and amateurs (ibid.). As Federman writes, Buddhism 'was textual, rationalistic, pragmatic, advocating a return to "original" forms, universal, and socially active' (Federman 2015, 554; see also Baumann 2002).

The interpretation of Buddhism as uniquely compatible with scientific method and theory was quickly taken up as one influence among many in ongoing processes of religious reform in Asia (Masuzawa 2005, 308). Informed by complex local political and social histories, reformers incorporated modernist trends in an evolving international dialogue conducted across networks of Buddhist knowledge (Cassaniti 2016; McDaniel 2011). Reformers in Asia presented Buddhism as a form of beneficial scientific rationality and exercise, and thereby invoked religious pluralism in its applicability (if Buddhism is a philosophy that transcends all religions then it is of benefit to all those who practise it, irrespective of their lower-level religious beliefs); as McMahan notes (2008, 90),

> While all historical religious traditions in their encounter with modernity have had to reinterpret doctrines in light of science's dominance, symbolic capital, tremendous transformative effects on the world, and unsurpassed legitimacy in establishing 'what is the case,' perhaps no major tradition has attempted to ally itself with scientific discourse more boldly than Buddhism.

Asian reformers and European scholars highlighted a contrast between arcane mysticism and applied science or rationalism, the underlying logic of which is 'that the Buddha himself taught a rationalist, empirically based, psychological, and ethical doctrine that was free of "superstition", largely compatible with modern science, and was preserved in the Pali suttas' (McMahan 2008, 65; see also McMahan 2004). Reflecting what Hallisey has referred to as (2014, 94) as practices of 'intercultural mimesis', this projection of modern values either overlooked or reinterpreted Buddhist cosmological principles that were not compatible with a proto-scientific worldview. Subsequent reformers interpreted those aspects of Buddhism that were not compatible with a rationalist-empiricist logic (for example, rituals, worship of the Buddha and deities, protective practices, realms of existence beyond the human) as either cultural pollutions masking the 'essence' of 'pure' Buddhism, or as psychological states, thus either detraditionalising or demythologising the Buddhist pantheon and reducing gods and spirits to moments of consciousness.

In Europe, emphasis on moral rationality was complemented by a contrastive interpretation of Buddhism and 'Eastern' religion more broadly. Late

Victorian and early Edwardian fascination with the occult, magic and spiritual experience informed orientalist interpretations of Buddhism as a repository of perennialist wisdom. At a time when discussion of the world's major religions and 'Eastern' sacred texts had become a staple of European cultural life, Buddhism was interpreted as a means of accessing perennial ancient wisdom for the benefit of humanity, reflecting broader Romantic reactions to Enlightenment thinking. Friedrich Max Müller, who held the first chair of comparative philology at Oxford, published his *Sacred Books of the East* in the 1870s, making religious texts from Asia available to the British public, and Edwin Arnold's sympathetic representation of the Buddha's life in *The Light of Asia* (2009 [1879]) seized the Victorian imagination. In reaction to widespread concerns about the alienating, stultifying or atomising effects of modern life, Buddhism was recast as an exotic 'Eastern' counterpoint to the ills of 'Western' society, through which Europeans could tap into Asian spiritual traditions. The destabilisation wrought by the social and technological shifts of the European Enlightenment and the scientific revolution, in forms such as bureaucratisation and the transformation of labour structures, was met by trends of increasing Romanticism and subjectification (see Taylor 1989). The Romantics proposed creative acts as a way of enlarging identity and recognising one's interconnectedness with others. Feelings of oneness or connection sought in nature and religious experience were understood to be a source of values and a means for redressing the worst effects of modernity, and the romantic tension between individualism and universalism—in which the ego is a lower form of self, masking higher forms of interrelatedness—was reflected in the British interest in Buddhism.

This association was developed in the work of the Theosophical Society, arguably the most famous esoteric group in late Victorian Britain. Founded by Henry Steel Olcott (1832–1904) and Helena P. Blavatsky (1877–1891), theosophy stemmed from a spiritualist movement committed to bridging the divide between the human and spirit worlds and investigating supernatural phenomena, mesmerism and mediumship, and arguably served as 'a romantic foil to the rationalism of the scholars' (Batchelor 1994, 270). Olcott and Blavatsky believed that perennial ancient wisdom underlay all religions, and they identified Buddhism as the best example of this primordial tradition, becoming the first Westerners to formally convert to Buddhism in 1880 (Prothero 1996). They promoted a universalist vision of the dharma in Europe and America, and to Buddhists in India and Ceylon, drawing on elements of Enlightenment philosophy, Romantic thought and late nineteenth-century occultism.[3] Owen argues (2004, 22) that the Theosophical Society had such wide appeal in Britain because it offered ordinary men and women the possibility of accessing esoteric knowledge. What marked the Theosophical Society as 'occult', and accounted for much of its appeal in Britain, was its members' belief that there exists a hidden body of revelatory knowledge, a secret tradition, that is transmitted by an enlightened group of spiritual masters called the 'mahatmas' (McMahan 2004, 908). Alfred Percy Sinnett, a member of the Anglo-Indian elite, published his influential work *Esoteric Buddhism* in 1883 after being impressed by Blavatsky's skills as a medium and her ability to receive messages from the mahatmas. Returning to England, Sinnett was highly influential in the 1880s and is in part responsible for the strong association of the Theosophical Society with 'the East' (Owen 2004, 31). Similarly, Carlton Massey, a barrister and Christian spiritualist, established the first branch of the London Theosophical Society in 1878 after meeting Blavatsky and Olcott in America (see Owen 2004). Drawing from Hinduism and Buddhism, theosophy reworked concepts of karma and reincarnation into an evolutionary theory of humankind and the universe. 'Theosophical teachings therefore lay great stress on individual evolution and perfection, and offer an all-encompassing account of individual existence in a living, meaningful universe' (ibid., 34).

Buddhism and Psychology

These two interpretations of Buddhism, as a rational and ethicised religion and as a medium for Romantic and perennialist oneness, arguably combined in the growing fascination with psychology as simultaneously scientific and spiritual. In Britain interest in both Buddhism and psychology was informed by popular fascination with both scientific verifiability and human potential. As Thomson writes of the unprecedented popular interest in psychological knowledge at that time (2006, 8), psychology was 'for some a science whose ambitions had to be contained if it was to justify [. . . its] status; for others a key to making sense of everything, a source of values for the new age, even a new way of reconciling science with religion'. Popular psychology movements arose motivated by excitement about the possibilities of human potential, informed by an idea that full self-realisation could be attained through accessing and mobilising the hidden powers of the mind (for a comparative case in America, see Albanese 2007).

One of the earliest iterations of Buddhism as a 'science of the mind' came from British Pali scholars Thomas W. Rhys Davids (1843–1922) and

Caroline A. F. Rhys Davids (1857–1942). The former founded the Pali Text Society in 1881 and was committed to the study of Buddhist texts. Reflecting the historicism of the time, he aimed to reveal the objective meaning of texts by applying the critical methods of 'scientific history' and de-emphasised ritual and religious practice (see Hallisey 2014). However, in the first decades of the twentieth century this framing found an unusual kinship with Romantic interpretations of Buddhism in a psychological register. The idea of Buddhism as a 'science of the mind' echoed interpretations of religion as pragmatic and experiential in essence, aimed at curing the ills of the human mind. For example, the American psychologist William James's seminal work *The Varieties of Religious Experience* (1902) shared in the Romantic desire to heal the 'divided self'. In his development of the psychology of religion, James sought to bracket truth claims concerning the content of religious experiences: while scientific observers may be able to observe that religious experience produces a feeling of oneness, they should not take this as proof that the cosmos is in fact one. Instead, the experience ought to be judged by its effects on the personality, in the pursuit of personal integration. This valorisation of experience found kinship with perennialist presentations of Buddhism: that there are many paths to the same reality, and one can thus select elements from different traditions on one's journey of self-discovery. James invited Thomas W. Rhys Davids to lecture at Harvard University on 'Buddhism: Its History and Literatures' in 1894/1895 (Stanley 2012, 202) and the Sri Lankan reformer Anagarika Dharmapala, during his third visit to America (1902–1904), attended a lecture given by James at Harvard. When James noticed him in the audience, he called Dharmapala to the front: 'Take my chair,' he is reported to have said, 'and I shall sit with my students. You are better equipped to lecture on psychology than I am.' Dharmapala gave a short lecture on Buddhist teaching, and James is reported to have remarked to his students, 'This is the psychology everybody will be studying twenty-five years from now' (Sangharakshita 2008 [1952], 35).[4]

Religion became newly valued as a quest for a feeling-experience, with religious doctrines being reinterpreted as a response to that experience. Such logics are reflected in the development of popular psychology movements in Britain in the first decades of the twentieth century, with their emphasis on spontaneity, self-fulfilment and authenticity. Propagated through clubs, correspondence courses and advice literature, movements such as the Practical Psychology movement, New Thought movement, spiritualism and Pelmanism[5] were all characterised by an extreme suspicion of conventional medicine, and an emphasis on self-improvement through the interrelationship between the mind, body and spirit (Thomson 2006, 22). Such movements were optimistic about being on the cusp of a new era of human power as a result of psychological self-improvement (ibid., 37). For example, the focus of Pelmanism and the practical psychology movement was pragmatic, and their popularity was matched by interest in more mystical understandings of psychology propagated through the London Psycho-therapeutic Society, linking psychology to the lineage of occult, spiritualist and mesmerist thought and practice (ibid., 26). Thus, by the start of the twentieth century, Britain had a widespread culture of psychological thinking that was informed by a model of the mind as a site of possibility and power. In the years following the First World War, the idea was well established that psychology was of central importance in life and could be put into practice by British people, thereby adding to the nation's mental efficiency, and could 'help the British brain' regain 'its position of predominance' (ibid., 23). Thomson argues that the popular psychology of this era inherited what we might see as a kind of secular, human-centred spirituality (ibid., 45). It was driven by excitement that man was at the threshold of discovering a greater psychological self: by uncovering the hidden potential of the mind, health, happiness and success would follow.

Despite Victorian interest in Buddhism, however, hardly any British people had converted to the religion (see Almond 1988, 36). Furthermore, British interest in Buddhism did not extend to meditation practice. While non-Buddhist forms of meditation, such as those based on Ignatius of Loyola's *Spiritual Exercises*, had become popular in Roman Catholic and Anglo-Catholic circles mid-century, Buddhist meditation did not occupy a central place in nineteenth-century European philological accounts, in part because of the intellectual bias of early European scholars, more concerned with religious texts than practice, but also because they simply did not have access to lived practice. In 1910 Rhys Davids published his translation of the Mahāsatipatthāna Sutta (titled *The Setting Up of Mindfulness*) (Federman 2015, 559). But Federman conjectures (2015, 558) that the Rhys Davidses and their contemporaries could not have had contact with anyone who practised what we might call Buddhist meditation. The early associations between meditation, magic and occult practices meant that meditation did not become the focus of Buddhism enthusiasts until much later (ibid., 557). Thus, meditation was either understood as an occult practice associated with cultivating powers, or it was sidelined in favour of a rationalist interpretation of Buddhism as philosophy and morality.[6] In Asia at the time, meditation was considered to be an advanced and perilous discipline, strongly associated with divine powers and inaccessible to the laity (see Cook 2010a, 33; Gombrich and Obeyesekere 1988, 237; Spiro 1970, 51). Gombrich and Obeyesekere (1988) tell us that the Buddhist reformer Anagarika Dharmapala taught himself to mediate from a manuscript of the Mahāsatipatthāna Sutta and that there were no meditation teachers in Ceylon (Sri Lanka) at the turn of the century. Thus, 'meditation' came to Britain as a concept, rather than a practice, which drew on the established Victorian meaning of meditation as 'contemplation'.

Meditation in Britain

Meditation only began to catch on in Britain after the First World War, with the establishment of the Buddhist Lodge of the Theosophical Society founded by Christmas Humphreys in 1924 (Oldmeadow 2004, 91), which included a practically oriented emphasis on meditation as an 'attempt to live the fundamental principles of Buddhism' (Humphreys 1937, 53). In reaction to the growing sense of helplessness in the face of political and economic uncertainty, the horrors of war and the decline of Christian faith, meditation provided a means for inner work and spiritual strength. Humphreys, who had turned away from his own Christian faith after losing his older brother in the war, understood the difference between Theosophy and Buddhism to be one of emphasis, rather than content, and the perennialism of the theosophists was echoed in his writing: 'Buddha's Teaching was not born from a spiritual vacuum, but was an expression of some portion of that Gupta Vidya, "the accumulated Wisdom of the ages", which antedates all known religions' (Humphreys 2012 [1974], 23). In 1926 the British branch of Dharmapala's Maha Bodhi Society was established and Humphreys became president of the Buddhist Lodge, newly re-established as the British Buddhist Society. Interest in meditation began to expand and meetings were held at the Buddhist Society several times a week.

Meditation was alternatively understood as a psychological and rational 'science' and as a practice for the transcendence of the intellect (Federman 2015, 554). Psychoanalysis was the first school of psychological thought to incorporate a sustained engagement with Buddhist teachings and practices, but it was arguably more influential in America than in Britain (see Helderman 2019). Interest in Freud and psychoanalysis amongst the British intelligentsia in the first decades of the twentieth century was complemented by excitement about 'Eastern mysticism' and alternative psychological approaches (Thomson 2006, 103). Jung describes the alarming moment of his break with Freud, when Freud asked him to promise never to abandon Freudian sexual theory but to make of it a 'dogma', an 'unshakable bulwark against the black tide of mud of occultism' (Jung 1961, 150; see Rose 1999). In 1927 Jung wrote a preface to *Bar do thos grol* (*The Tibetan Book of the Dead*) in which he interpreted the *bar dos* (the intermediate states between lives) as levels of the unconscious and Buddhist deities as expressions of universal archetypes in the collective unconsciousness, thereby demythologising the Tibetan pantheon of gods and spirits and rendering them facets of the mind. In Britain, Jung's influence on intellectuals such as Aldous and Julian Huxley underpinned their commitment to an idea of psychosocial evolution as a new basis for humanism. It was thought that the psychological evolution of the individual human consciousness would lead to a new age of consciousness.

By the 1930s in Britain, meditation was predominantly thought of as a technique for controlling one's own mind (Federman 2015, 566). The decade saw a series of articles giving practical advice on how to meditate, and meditation instruction being given at the Lodge every second Monday evening. Public talks on how to meditate were also scheduled at the Maha Bodhi Society in London. It was in the interwar period that 'stress' emerged, on both sides of the Atlantic, as a focus for preoccupations with the harmful effects of modern lifestyles (Jackson 2013, 53). Mundane aspects of everyday life—domestic demands, the strain of work, urbanisation and consumerism—were increasingly causally linked to a rise in stress-related disorders (ibid., 188) and relaxation techniques were promoted as a way to live happier and healthier lives (Nathoo 2019, 10). While early twentieth-century formulations of nervous disorders conceptualised stress as an external agent that generated the psychological and physical symptoms of distress, it became increasingly common in the interwar years for clinicians and popular commentators to understand the rise of organic and psychological disease in terms of maladjustment or a faulty adaptation to the environment (Jackson 2013, 17). The relationship between social conditions, personal resilience and health became the focus of psychologists and physiologists who sought to identify strategies for coping with the stress of modern life (ibid., 187). In the work of people such as the endocrinologist Hans Selye (1907–1982) and psychologist Richard Lazarus (1922–2002), emphasis began to shift from a focus on environment to the adoption of coping strategies to counter the effects of stress (ibid., 214). Relaxation techniques were established as increasingly medically supported practices for the mainstream British public. Nathoo (2019) demonstrates that in the 1930s relaxation was presented as a skill that could be learned, cultivated and applied for therapeutic effect, and relaxation teachings were disseminated to a wide audience, notably through popular books, antenatal instruction and speech therapy. In Britain, the injunction 'You must relax' was taken up by participants in relaxation classes looking to manage the stresses of daily life.

By the 1930s interest in spiritual transcendence and supernormal psychological power was fading in favour of psychology as an everyday assistance, which addressed specific problems rather than general principles (Thomson 2006, 48). Moreover, the idea of psychological subjectivity was figured in Britain, at the prospect of a second world war, in contrast to the problems of war and political extremism of other European nations, both of which were understood as resulting from the human potential for violence. In the 1930s psychological ideas about innate aggression appealed to left-wing audiences, who found in this framing a way of countering the prevailing Marxist view that the international situation could be explained in purely economic terms. For example, attacks on Jews and Communists were understood to stem from a 'scapegoat motive' as an expression of human aggression. By recognising and controlling this, the problems of war could be addressed (Thomson 2006, 221–22). Here, then, the link between democracy, peace and mental health was made explicitly British. As Thomson writes, in British people's self-representations, 'British national character emerged, implicitly if not explicitly, as the embodiment of psychological health' (ibid., 224). This contrasted with other nations, with regard to which aggression and war were framed as symptomatic of psychological character, as in the case of the rise of Fascism (see, e.g., Reich 1970 [1946]). Britain's political and psychological health were understood to be mutually reinforcing.[7]

By the start of the 1940s, a popular discourse had developed of meditation as spiritual work which touched the deeper domains of the psyche that were inaccessible to rational thinking. The increasing popularity of psychoanalysis in Britain reframed the meaning of meditation as a technique for accessing the hidden realms of the psyche in order to reveal these in a process of personal transformation. Psychoanalysis developed as a method for exploring the unconscious forces which drive human behaviour in ways that rationality could not control, as evidenced in the destruction wrought by war, and meditation began to be associated with psychological therapy as a form of medicine for the mind. A development from the 1930s theme of 'mind-control', the turn to the psyche offered healing from the effects of social and political instability. Federman writes (2015, 570) of the British association between meditation and psychological exploration in the 1940s that '[m]editation came to be talked about as a spiritual medicine for cleaning a psyche which is clogged by waste matter. The practice of such meditation transcends rationality and its limited powers. It goes deeper into the hidden realms of the self in order to transform it.'

As psychoanalysis became popular in Britain, the idea of the psyche as irrational and dangerous came to rival an emphasis on rationality and ethics. At the same time, national and psychological responses to the Second World War incorporated understandings of resilience, in terms of, for example, 'character', fortitude and 'grit', as the inner attributes of the subject. As Chandler writes (2014, 10), 'Britain was resilient because the superior firepower of the German air force failed to achieve its aim of defeating and demoralising the British people during the Blitz'. The resilient subject was conceived of as capable of overcoming environmental challenges or oppressive social conditions through her inner strengths and capacities. In response to post-imperial decline, British self-representation held that Britain was able to 'bat above its weight' because of the 'bulldog' spirit of its people (ibid.).

The Development of Insight and Buddhism in Britain

From the 1950s onwards, a multiplicity of Buddhist groups began to establish themselves in Britain through the development of both monastic centres and lay groups. Bluck notes that, while each had its own history, Buddhist traditions and sub-traditions were informed by rapid changes in British culture, including greater socioeconomic mobility, the declining influence of the church and increasing interest in 'oriental' religions, the expansion of higher education, a newly permissive youth culture, British perception of the Chinese invasion of Tibet and the American war in Vietnam (Bluck 2008, 10; for comparative European cases, see Borup 2008; Plank 2010; Prohl 2014). Prior to the 1950s, the figure of the European Buddhist was conceived of as 'a rational, detached person who intellectually purifies himself (seldom herself) from the root defilements of ignorance, hatred, and lustfulness' (Baumann 2002, 91). During the 1960s, a shift occurred in the way in which British people engaged with Buddhism. They increasingly wanted to *experience* Buddhism through meditation as they began to look for alternative life orientations, and found in meditation simultaneously a rational tool for psychological development and a method for transcending the rational mind. Informed by a broader culture of 'spiritual seeking' and an eclectic mix of traditions, gurus, devotion and psychology, increasing numbers of British youths were travelling in Asia on the 'hippy trail' and seeking out Buddhist professionals at newly established monastic centres in Britain. As Baumann notes (ibid., 92), 'The romantic yearning for wholeness and originality was sought—again—in the East.' Meditation became a therapeutic practice, a means for self-cultivation through a sense of oneness or wonder in daily life, understood as an antidote to the materialist implications of science.

British interest in meditation was informed by an emerging mass lay meditation movement in Asia. Beginning in the early twentieth century, an unprecedented lay meditation movement grew rapidly in Theravada Buddhist countries. Drawing on the teaching of the Mahāsatipatthāna Sutta (The greater discourse on the four foundations of mindfulness), reformist monks instigated a modern meditation movement that claimed its antecedent roots in the canonical word of the Buddha (for a history of mass meditation in Burma, see Braun 2013). Whereas previously, received wisdom held that lay people could not achieve the concentration required for meditative insight, and thus practice was not appropriate in their mundane lives, reformist meditation masters such as Ledi Sayadaw (1846–1923), U Ba Khin (1899–1971) and Mahasi Sayadaw (1904–1982) argued that insight (*vipassanā*) meditation techniques required only a minimal level of concentration. Mahasi Sayadaw's radical claim was that liberating insight did not require advanced concentration (*samatha*) or the experience of meditative absorption (*jhana*). Mahasi emphasised instead *sati* (Pali; Sanskrit *smṛti*), understood as moment-to-moment awareness of whatever sensory object arises in the flow of consciousness. In south and south-east Asia, *vipassanā* meditation was presented to the laity as a way to find relief from worldly concerns by enjoying the benefits of meditative exercise.[8] Southeast Asian urban meditation movements of the 1970s responded to an environment that involved Western education and scientific ideology, the meditation groups modelling themselves as 'research centres' (Van Esterik 1977). The new centrality of meditation led to the revival, democratisation and popularisation of canonical meditation techniques, made available in meditation centres.

The term 'mindfulness' seems to have first been used by T. W. Rhys Davids in his early translation of the Buddhist term *sati*.[9] Mindfulness came to be defined as a form of awareness, de-emphasising variegated definitions of the notion in earlier Buddhist accounts in which aspects of remembering, recalling, reminding and presence of mind predominated (Gethin 2011; Sharf 2017). In *The Heart of Buddhist Meditation* the German-born Sri-Lankan monk Nyanaponika Thera (1901–1994), interpreted mindfulness as 'bare attention'. Mindfulness, he argued, is not a 'mystical' state: 'In its elementary manifestation, known under the term "attention", it is one of the cardinal functions of consciousness without which there cannot be perception of any object at all' (Nyanaponika Thera 1962, 24).

Nyanaponika contrasted 'bare attention' with habits of judging from the perspective of self-interest: rather than seeing things as they are from a position of disinterested appraisal, people habitually view objects 'in the light of added subjective judgements' (ibid., 32–34). Nyanaponika understood mindfulness as a quality of awareness which could act as a counter to the constant reinforcement of habitual mental patterns (Gethin 2011, 267). This 'bare attention' was newly presented as central to *vipassanā* meditation, which was itself newly promoted as the 'heart' of Buddhist meditation practice. Mindfulness began to emerge as a form of non-judgemental, direct observation of mind and body in the present moment, in ways that would lead to 'insight' (*vipassanā*), broadly understood.

The influence of Asian migrant populations on the perception of Buddhism in Europe gained in prominence in the 1960s and 1970s as Buddhist migrant communities began to form (Baumann 2002, 86), and British people increasingly looked to meditation as a way of experiencing Buddhism. While in the context of the US, ideas about irrational forms of immigrant religious practice prevailed and immigrant Buddhist temples and mindfulness centres were clearly demarcated (see Hickey 2010), Baumann reports (2002) that in Britain the same racialised distinctions were not established. *Vipassanā* and Zen courses proliferated and Baumann tells us (ibid., 92) that they were often booked up well in advance. British awareness of a wide range of traditions and practices had grown, and a close association was made between New Age movements and Buddhism: both were interpreted as sharing the utopianism and perennialism of Theosophist heritage (Cush 1996, 206) and were associated with meditation, human potential, environmentalism, and peace (ibid., n. 195). In the 1970s the newly formed Insight Meditation tradition was advanced and propagated in the UK by meditation teachers including Christina Feldman, John Peacock and Martine and Stephen Batchelor, and in America by teachers including Jack Kornfield, Joseph Goldstein and Sharon Salzberg. Now world-renowned, each of these teachers had spent time in Asia, many taking ordination as monastics, and returned to the UK and US to teach meditation, establishing now famous meditation centres such as Gaia House (founded 1976) in the UK, and the Insight Meditation Society (IMS; founded 1975) in the States (see Cadge 2005). Echoing the teachings of Nyanaponika

Thera, and foreshadowing much of the interpretation of mindfulness that was to come, Jack Kornfield wrote (1977, 13),

The most direct way to understand our life situation, who we are and how we operate, is to observe with a mind that simply notices all events equally. This attitude of non-judgmental, direct observation allows all events to occur in a natural way. By keeping attention in the present moment, we can see more and more clearly the true characteristics of our mind and body process.

Meditation was increasingly represented as a method for psychological development which accorded with Enlightenment ideas of the perfectibility of man through moral reflection, self-observation and control of the passions (see McMahan 2008, 203), but this was not at the expense of a more Romantic interpretation of the practice as a method for direct experience of authentic interrelatedness.

Mindfulness and Mental Health

Although, as we have seen, Buddhism had been interpreted as a rational, science-compatible religion since the end of the nineteenth century, it was not until very recently that it became itself the focus of scientific studies. As McMahan and Braun report, the number of publications on 'mindfulness' in scientific journals in the entire decade of the 1980s totalled thirteen. In the 1990s this number grew to ninety-two; while 674 articles were published on mindfulness in 2015 alone (McMahan and Braun 2017, 1–2). The definitions of mindfulness that inform contemporary psychological studies have much in common with Nyanaponika Thera's earlier understanding of mindfulness as 'bare attention' and the methods of the Insight Tradition developed in Britain and America. For example, Bishop et al. (2004, 232) define mindfulness as 'a kind of nonelaborative, nonjudgmental, present-centered awareness in which each thought, feeling, or sensation that arises in the attentional field is acknowledged and accepted as it is'. Similarly, an understanding of mindfulness as a non-elaborative choiceless awareness is echoed in Kabat-Zinn's much referenced definition (1994, 4): 'paying attention in a particular way: on purpose, in the present moment, and nonjudgmentally'.

Without doubt, the most influential and thoroughly researched development of meditation as a therapeutic tool is the Mindfulness-Based Stress

Reduction (MBSR) programme (see Braun 2017; McMahan 2008; Wilson 2014). Developed by Jon Kabat-Zinn in 1979, MBSR began as an outpatient service at the hospital of the University of Massachusetts. As well as working at the medical school as a researcher and gross anatomy instructor, Kabat-Zinn had practised Tibetan *dzogchen*, taught yoga and become a certified dharma teacher at the Cambridge Zen Center in Cambridge, Massachusetts. Towards the end of a two-week meditation retreat at the Insight Meditation Society (IMS) in Barre, Massachusetts, led by two British Insight Meditation teachers, Christopher Titmuss and Christina Feldman, Kabat-Zinn experienced a 'vision' of MBSR (Kabat-Zinn 2011, 287):

> I saw in a flash not only a model that could be put into place, but also the long-term implications of what might happen if the basic idea was sound and could be implemented in one test environment—namely that it would spark new fields of scientific and clinical investigation, and would spread to hospitals and medical centres and clinics across the country and around the world, and provide right livelihood for thousands of practitioners.... after that retreat, I did have a better sense of what my karmic assignment might be.

MBSR was designed originally to help people with chronic pain and a range of conditions that were difficult to treat (Kabat-Zinn 2013 [1990]), drawing on a range of different traditions in a routinised eight-week course for outpatients. It drew largely on meditation techniques from the IMS Insight Meditation tradition (see Gilpin 2008, 238), but included body scan practices based on the teachings of the Burmese-Indian teacher S. N. Goenka, and mindful movement techniques stemming from hatha yoga (Braun 2017). Braun argues that a 'Zen sensibility' also pervades Kabat-Zinn's teaching, evidenced in his use of the vocabulary of non-doing and nonduality, the presentation of mindfulness through paradox and contradiction, and a sense of ineffability and a focus on the everyday (ibid., 181). This hybrid of Burmese, Zen and Tibetan traditions was synthesised through Kabat-Zinn's interpretation of the dharma in a universal register as the nature of experience revealed through mindful awareness. In the 1980s he was finding ways to articulate for professional and lay audiences what he identified as the origins and essence of Buddhist teachings (Kabat-Zinn 2011, 283):

> how the Buddha himself was not a Buddhist, how the word *Buddha* means one who has awakened, and how mindfulness, often spoken of as 'the heart

of Buddhist meditation', has little or nothing to do with Buddhism, per se, and everything to do with wakefulness, compassion, and wisdom. These are universal qualities of being human, precisely what the word *dharma*, is pointing to.

This framing reflects the earlier perennialist thought of the theosophists and transcendentalists,[10] in that it emphasises universal 'experience' prior to doctrine or tradition, but it does so in a way that naturalises both religion and psychological knowledge: the dharma can be explained in scientific terms. MBSR proved to be demonstrably effective in the reduction of pain, and scientific evidence for its efficacy became crucial to its popularity and uptake (Kabat-Zinn 1982). But, if science is the home ground of rationalism, in the development of MBSR it became imbued with a Romantic commitment to wonder and meaning: mindfulness was intended to 'rehumanise' science and modern life more generally (McMahan 2008, 213–14). Braun notes (2017, 174) that from the outset MBSR was intended to lead to transformative life experiences permeated with depth and value by drawing on bodily experience, results from empirical studies, American 'spirituality' and a range of Buddhist teachings. Participants on MBSR courses were encouraged to move from a reactive aversion to pain to a non-judgemental awareness and acceptance of the experience. This changed psychological engagement with localised pain had broader implications for experiences in life more generally. As Braun puts it (ibid., 175), in Kabat-Zinn's teaching, '[p]ain, mindfully observed, offers the charter opportunity to change one's relationship to all experience'. Braun argues that modern liberal Romantic ideas that highlight interiority, self-determination and an affinity for Asian thought, centring on the mind and its energetic movements, are reflected in contemporary articulations of mindfulness in America. The construction of a 'metaphysical Asia' (Albanese 2007, 330) drew on transcendentalist and spiritualist movements, a heritage of metaphysical religiosity that informed 'spiritual seeker culture' and the popularity of mindfulness (Braun 2017, 188). Echoing earlier transcendentalist principles of experience and ecumenicalism (see McMahan 2008, 165–68) spirituality became sedimented in secular contexts without requiring metaphysical commitment (see Bender 2010, 182–83). For example, Kabat-Zinn writes (1994, 5),

The key to this path which lies at the root of Buddhism, Taoism, and yoga, and which we also find in the work of people like Emerson, Thoreau, and Whitman, and in Native American wisdom, is an appreciation for the present moment and the cultivation of an intimate relationship with it through a continual attending to it with care and discernment.

Mindfulness, then, had come to reflect the Enlightenment values of moral striving and self-making, evidenced in the empirically measurable universal framework of the science of the mind, one which is invested with ethical value, meaning and purpose. As Braun writes (2017, 195), Kabat-Zinn's teaching 'stresses a naturalized sense of meaning, one that goes beyond Buddhism and is rooted in everyday experience—particularly painful experience. What is more, this experience is scientifically validated through empirical study.' The structuring of a disposition that is 'spiritual-but-not-religious' is naturalised through empirical emphasis on efficacy and utility, such that the 'spiritual' is reframed as depth and value in the everyday.

It was not until the development of Mindfulness-Based Cognitive Therapy (MBCT) in 1991 that mindfulness-based therapies began to impact healthcare significantly in Britain. Drawing inspiration from Mindfulness-Based Stress Reduction (MBSR) in America (see Braun 2017; McMahan 2008; Wilson 2014), MBCT was developed by Zindel Segal, John Teasdale and Mark Williams in Cambridge, UK, as a psychosocial intervention to address depressive relapse. By the 1980s and 1990s, depression was being identified as one of the major mental health problems facing the UK. Robust and effective interventions were being developed to treat people experiencing an episode of acute depression as either a psychobiological or a psychosocial disorder. However, beginning in the 1980s, an understanding began to emerge of depression as a recurring condition; it was becoming clear that people who had recovered from a depressive episode remained vulnerable to relapse. The concern was that Britain was on the cusp of a mental health crisis and that interventions that addressed the acute phase of depression were not enough; people who had recovered from distress faced serious challenges in maintaining their mental health, and a long-term approach to therapy was required. By the late 1980s psychopharmacological intervention began to be reframed as a prophylactic intervention, and maintenance antidepressant medication (m-ADM) for as long as three–five years was encouraged for those deemed to be most vulnerable to relapse. But for those people for whom antidepressants are not appropriate, an alternative was needed.

Originally, Segal, Teasdale and Williams set out to develop a maintenance form of cognitive therapy. People who had received cognitive therapy during acute depression proved less likely to experience depressive relapse. Segal et al.

began to explore the possibility that cognitive therapy had a long-term benefi-
cial effect, not because the content of thoughts about the self were changed,
but because the task itself changed the relationship that people had to thoughts
(Segal, Williams and Teasdale 2013, 36). John Teasdale, who had long practised
meditation, attended a Dharma Talk at the Oxford Buddhist Centre given by
Phra Ajharn Sumedho, the then head of the Thai forest tradition in the UK.
Ajharn Sumedho expounded on the Buddha's teaching of the Four Noble
Truths and Teasdale was struck by a parallel between Ajharn Sumedho's teaching that the causes of suffering lie in the ways in which one relates to experiences, rather than the experiences themselves, and the cognitive framework
for depressive relapse, in which emotional disorder results from the interpretations that are added to experience, rather than the experiences themselves
(Teasdale 2009). The cognitive framework of MBCT rests on the twin premise
that there is a cognitive component to depressive relapse and that people have
the capacity to learn ways of relating to their thoughts and feelings that will
enable them to maintain mental and emotional balance, even in the face of
challenging affective experiences. Evidence for the efficacy of MBCT, garnered
through randomised controlled trials (RCTs) and advanced statistical analysis, particularly meta-analyses, has spurred the adoption of MBCT in Britain,
and, by extension, the popularity of mindfulness. Three early RCTs concluded
that MBCT was equivalent to treatment as usual (TAU) and maintenance
antidepressants in the prevention of depressive relapse (Kuyken et al. 2008;
Ma and Teasdale 2004; Teasdale, Segal et al. 2000). As a direct result of these
findings, the National Institute for Health and Care Excellence (NICE) included MBCT as a key priority in its 2009 prevention strategy (Clause 8.10.8.1),
and MBCT was made available through the National Health Service (NHS)
for those most at risk of depressive relapse.

Buddhist-derived meditation practice was interpreted as universal and
compatible with cognitive psychology. As Williams and Kabat-Zinn write in
a co-authored paper (2011, 3),

Since Buddhist meditative practices are concerned with embodied awareness and the cultivation of clarity, emotional balance (equanimity) and
compassion, and since all of these capacities can be refined and developed
via the honing and intentional deployment of attention, the roots of Buddhist meditation practices are de facto universal.

Thus, mindfulness meditation was identified as the essence of Buddhism and
as a universally applicable practice. Simultaneously, Buddhism and science

were interpreted as equivalent epistemologies, dialogue between which would facilitate human flourishing. MBCT and MBSR were described as 'marriages' between a conceptual framework of cognitive psychology and quite intensive training in mindfulness meditation—a 'confluence of two powerful and potentially synergistic epistemologies' (ibid., 1). The 'intermixing of streams' was intended to benefit the world 'as long as the highest standards of rigor and empiricism native to each stream are respected and followed' (ibid., 3–4). Buddhism was interpreted as a universal ethic, or shared truth, which may be accessed through Buddhist teaching or practice but was not limited to it. Truth, then, in scientific and Buddhist practice, was understood to transcend specific cultural contexts or religious allegiances.[11]

MBCT was developed at a time of wider interest in preventative healthcare in the UK. Since the millennium, increasing emphasis has been placed on preventative medicine, patient empowerment and behaviour change, to encourage people to moderate behaviours linked to chronic illness and disease (see, e.g., Abraham and Michie 2008). Public mental health in Britain is increasingly focused on primary prevention approaches, which seek to stop mental health problems before they develop by encouraging mental resilience. Such primary prevention approaches to mental health are 'universal', in that they do not target populations specifically at risk but rather seek to benefit everyone in a community. As we will see in subsequent chapters, this shift from a focus on illness to health is reflected in the move from targeted interventions to everyday practices, echoing earlier iterations of interest in psychological potential. For example, six months before the launch of the *Mindful Nation* report, a national charity called the Mental Health Foundation (MHF) launched its campaign for mental health awareness week calling for a 'Prevention Revolution': a commitment to the prevention of mental health problems, tackling risks, intervening early and building resilience. Around the country, posters promoting mindfulness went up on billboards and bus shelters. Colourful advertisements exhorted commuters to 'Be Yourself', 'Be Connected', 'Be Here', 'Be Whole'. The legend was followed by a web link to BeMindful.co.uk and an encouragement to practice: 'Mindfulness is a way of managing your thoughts and feelings by focusing on the present, and can reduce stress and anxiety.'

In this emphasis on universal preventative healthcare and psychological resilience we see the intertwining of the threads of Romanticism and rationalism that informed earlier periods in this genealogy. Whereas earlier understandings of resilience framed the subject as actively conquering or passively

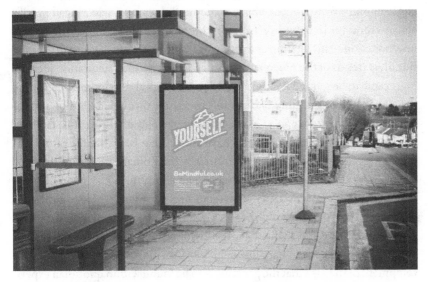

FIGURE 1. The Mental Health Foundation 'BeMindful' campaign, London,
May 2015. Image copyright Wellmind Health Limited.

coping with the external environment, resilience thinking has increasingly
drawn on a relationally embedded understanding of the subject in response
to intractable problems, such as mental health. Policy emphasis on mindfulness and resilience foregrounds the development of character traits and inner
capabilities of reflexivity and relational awareness. Mindfulness forms the basis
of a targeted intervention for specific goals, understood as a psychological
technique that is empirically validated. And it is promoted with the intention
of enabling practitioners to develop a deeper appreciation of daily activities
and a different engagement with life, thereby cultivating mental resilience. As
Chandler writes (2014, 11), '[i]n this process of self-reflective awareness, the
resilient subject emerges not as a secure subject but as a self-aware subject.'

Conclusion: The Rationalism and Romanticism
of the Present Moment

I hope to have shown that contemporary understandings of mindfulness as a
targeted psychological intervention and as a metaphysical technique for finding meaning and purpose in life have a long history. As we have seen, the currents of rationalism and Romanticism have circulated since the late nineteenth
century and these trends in intellectual and cultural thought have informed

contemporary British engagement with mindfulness as a scientifically verifiable method for living more 'fully'. In this chapter I have traced the British interpretation of meditation as a proto-scientific technique back to modernist Buddhist trends of the nineteenth century. In this period, meditation increasingly came to be framed as a method for psychological development, enabling the possibility of standing back from experience through a kind of 'radical reflexivity' (Taylor 1989, 163) in order to remake oneself through disciplined work. At the same time, I hope to have shown that British interest in Buddhism over this period was also motivated by the Romantic concern that modernity is leading to isolation, atomisation and ill-health. British people sought in Buddhism, and more latterly in meditation, a means of transcending the ills of modernity through an emphasis on a quality of engagement with 'ordinary' experience. This echoes what Charles Taylor has referred (1989, 211–304) to as the 'affirmation of ordinary life' in his work on modern subjectivity—a development of the idea that the good life is to be found within quotidian experience by engaging with it in a particular way. Thus, the contemporary British focus on preventative healthcare, mental resilience and meditation as a form of psychological support shares parallels, and sometimes direct links, with earlier movements.

The UK secretary of state's commitment to prophylactic psychological support at the *Mindful Nation* launch speaks to broader concerns about mental health and psychological vulnerability (see Cook 2018). In Britain, resilience has become 'the policy buzzword of choice' (Chandler 2014, 1; see chapter 6), presented as a solution to governance questions as wide-ranging as international development aid, the 'war on terror' and the prevalence of depression. Modern life is identified as leading to stress and illness, and forms of psychological support are required in the face of adversity. Mindfulness as a technique for encouraging psychological resilience is invested with a series of nested universalisms: the characterisation of human psychology as driven by flaws in cognition, the potential for psychological training to address the deleterious effects of modernity, the ability of scientific investigation to reveal the empirical efficacy of meditation and the phenomenology of a Romantic 'fullness' accessible through practice. What I hope to have shown is that changing patterns in British psychology and Buddhism do not reveal a deep subjectivity that transcends historical determination. Rather, each of these universalisms is constituted in and constitutive of broader historical and political contexts. Whereas twenty-first-century political interest is focused on mental health and resilience, earlier interventions focused on concepts of human potential, esoteric knowledge, mind training, practical psychology, anxiety and stress. This reveals that the excitement about the potential of psychology to support ordinary life is influenced in no small part by the social relationships from which it arises. The intention to cultivate psychological resilience through engagement with mindfulness practices saturates it with new qualities and meanings. In response to the challenges of a complex world, psychological resilience is thought to be achieved through the cultivation of character traits and capabilities of self-reflection and metacognition, informing the relational interaction between the subject and the external world.

The history of British engagement with Buddhism and psychology is steeped in the tensions that characterised nineteenth- and twentieth-century Britain: tensions between rationalist moves for empirical certainty and the Romantic call for meaning and experience, the development of psychology as a discipline and British skittishness about professional authority, the desire for the 'wisdom' of 'the East' and the novelty of progress, optimism about human potential and dystopian concerns about the consequences of modernity, the desire to live fully and the need to prevent illness. It highlights that the influence of psychological culture has been a constituent source of subjectivity in Britain in different ways since at least the nineteenth century, that contemporary interest in the intermixing of 'Eastern' and 'Western' ideas enjoys a long precedent, and that this is not the first time that concern over the effects of modernity has led to calls for renewed engagement with 'ordinary' life. If the 'present moment' is having its moment, it is not for the first time.

In the next chapter, I turn to mindfulness as a psychosocial therapeutic intervention for the prevention of depressive relapse. I examine three different forms of learning (cognitive, metacognitive and attitudinal) by which practitioners seek to relate to themselves and their experiences in order to prevent a relapse into depression and to support their mental health. I show that changes in the categorisation of depression are incorporated into people's experiences of themselves and their efforts to live well, as psychological categories are responded to through culturally shaped practices.

2

Depression, Optimism and Metacognition

BECKY DESCRIBES her relationship with herself as 'punishing'. She is in her mid-thirties, white, single and middle-class. She lives in the south-west of England and works as a freelance writer. Becky never self-identified as someone who has depression, though she thinks now that she must have done so for much of her adult life. When she was down, she would find ways to keep herself away from other people, making excuses to them and telling herself that she was too busy to see anyone. When her mood was at its lowest, she couldn't move. She couldn't open her post or respond to emails. Mess would mount up around the house, and for Becky the piles of unopened mail felt like a shaming testimony to her inertia. She would admonish herself, 'Bloody well sort it out. Pull yourself together,' frustrated by what she saw as ongoing personal failure. During these times she periodically thought about killing herself.

Becky knew that there were times when she felt more well than at others; sometimes her mental state put limits on her ability to do things, and sometimes it involved suicidal thoughts. She interpreted these not as symptoms of depression, but as a personal failure ('bloody well sort it out'). If at times she might have met the criteria for a mental health diagnosis, she only self-identified as someone with depression after years of low periods when her mental health was, as she put it, 'as bad as it's ever been'. In desperation, she spoke about her suicidal thoughts to her GP, who insisted that she start taking antidepressants. Becky hated this idea and persuaded her doctor to give her a little time to find an alternative, knowing that she would have little option but to take the medication if she couldn't find anything else to help. One of the things that she found was a nearby Mindfulness-Based Cognitive Therapy (MBCT) course, and she enrolled.

In this chapter I consider the consequences of the recent reframing of depression as a relapsing or recurring condition in Britain. I focus on MBCT courses, such as the one that Becky took, which are intended to prevent the relapse of what is called a 'major depressive episode' (MDE). I draw on two and a half years' participant observation on an MBCT therapist training course and an eight-week MBCT course for people with a history of depression and interviews with participants once they had completed both courses, and I refer to the specific details of an MBCT course on which I was a participant observer in May 2015. Through examining the structured learning process of the eight-week MBCT course, I demonstrate that mental health is now thought of as something that can be cultivated, both in the prevention of psychological disorder and as a positive component of healthy living.

An important chorus of social scientific work has built up over the last half-century that has critically evaluated the causes of suffering and the diagnostic category of 'depression'. Anthropologists have demonstrated in compelling ways that European and American psychiatric diagnoses are culturally constituted categories, and that applying them in diverse contexts may mask the complexity of culturally varied experiences of human suffering. In their seminal work *Culture and Depression* (1985), Kleinman and Good highlighted the fact that there are important differences in the experience and expression of depression-like symptoms in different places, demonstrating variation in the cultural organisation of what we often simply term 'depression'. They and their contributors revealed alternative idioms for depression-like experiences and culture-specific explanatory models for depressive disorder (see for example, Good and Good 1982; Good, Good and Moradi 1985; Keyes 1985; Kleinman 1982; Kleinman and Kleinman 1985; Lutz 1985; Marsella 1978; 1985; Schieffelin 1985). This scholarship challenged the assumption that psychiatric diagnostic criteria are somehow 'culture-free', thereby calling into question the applicability of 'depression' as a diagnostic category, and highlighting the cultural construction of psychiatric diagnostic categories and the fact that they may therefore change over time (see also Benedict 1934, Littlewood 1980; Littlewood and Dein 1995; Littlewood and Lipsedge 1987; 1997; White and Marsella 1982).[1]

Over the same period, anthropological analyses of depression have been influenced by broader trends in the social sciences. Scholars have repeatedly warned that psychology and psychiatry transform social and political problems into individual, biological or psychological concerns (see Cooper 1967; Ingleby 1980; Laing 1969; Szasz 1961). The first wave of medical anthropologists theorised medicine in broadly ideological terms, understanding medical practice, intervention and 'responsibility' as reproducing dominant power structures (see Zola 1972). This informed important work that analysed suffering through political, social and cultural frameworks (see Biehl 2005; Kirmayer 1991; Lutz 1985; Scheper-Hughes 1988).[2] Depression was theorised not as a psychiatric disorder but as a breakdown of community, '*a normal response to pathological social structures*' (Karp 1996, 80; italics in original), the implication being that we should address the inequities of social structures rather than pathologise appropriate responses to them.

The tension remains between social scientific critique and psychiatric categories. Kleinman and Good (1985), and those that followed them, were right to highlight that symptoms serve as the criteria for depressive illness and, given that symptoms vary significantly across cultures, establishing the cross-cultural validity of the category of 'depression' is challenging. It is certainly the case that the social meanings of the symptoms of a syndrome are crucial to diagnosis and treatment, that the categorisation of depressive disorders may not be sufficient to characterise the variance and breadth of symptomology, suffering and meaning, and that psychopathology may cut across existing diagnostic entities (Kirmayer 1991, 27). But at the same time, as Kleinman himself has pointed out, the primary mental disorders—depression among them—are identifiable worldwide (Kleinman 1988, 41) and a major cause of disability (see Kleinman 2004, 951). Furthermore, the tension between psychological and social causation remains present in debates about depression. While we cannot underestimate the important work that critical social scientific scholarship has done in highlighting the structural conditions that contribute to depression, depression cannot be accounted for *exclusively* as a problem of political, social or economic inequality. As Martin argues (2006, 151), 'Depression can be "normal", in the sense of an understandable and expected response to harmful social structures, and yet have pathological aspects that disrupt our ability to carry on with our lives. And we cannot wait until community problems are solved before dealing with suffering.' Depression is repeatedly revealed to be a complicated and multi-causal syndrome, one informed by physical, psychological, economic, cultural, social, structural and political factors, to say nothing of social equality and mobility. Bringing depression under control in its major or acute stages is neither quick nor easy, and those who claim a unitary cause or cure are often naive—or selling something (see Ecks 2005).

As we saw in the last chapter, MBCT was developed by Zindel Segal, John Teasdale and Mark Williams in Cambridge, UK, as a psychosocial

intervention for the prevention of depressive relapse, in response to the changing characterisation of depression as a relapsing or recurring condition. In
earlier nosologies, depression had been characterised as an acute, circumstantial or episodic condition that affected the patient, who, through engagement
with psychodynamic or psychopharmaceutical treatment, would return to full
health. But this has changed since the 1980s. Researchers found that severe
episodes of depression left a residual or latent vulnerability to relapse. Numerous studies estimated that at least 50 per cent of people who had experienced
an initial episode of depression would have at least one subsequent episode.
The likelihood of relapse in people who had experienced two or more episodes
increased to 70–80 per cent (Keller et al. 1983; Keller et al. 1992). Rather than
being understood as an acute short-term condition, depression was reframed
as an increase in long-term vulnerability, and a history of depression was to be
understood as a risk factor for chronic or recurring illness in healthy people.
While diagnostic categories are necessarily reductive classifications of human
suffering, they interact with people's understanding of themselves and their
experiences. In this new framing, depression became a condition to be treated,
a latent vulnerability in people who were well, and a predictor for future
episodes. And, as we saw in the last chapter, in the 1980s long-term pharmacological interventions were encouraged for those most at risk of depressive
relapse.[3]

The development of MBCT was informed by a reclassification of depression as a relapsing condition that can be addressed through psychosocial training. This led to transformations in both the 'meaning' of 'depression' and the
therapeutic interventions with which people engage. As we saw in chapter 1,
Segal, Teasdale and Williams set out originally to develop a maintenance form
of cognitive therapy. Cognitive therapy is focused on identifying negative beliefs, thoughts and attitudes that depressed people hold regarding themselves
and on changing the content of those thoughts. People who had received
cognitive therapy during acute depression proved less likely to experience
depressive relapse. Segal and his colleagues began to explore the possibility
that cognitive therapy had a long-term beneficial effect not because the content of thoughts about the self were changed, but because the task itself
changed the relationship that patients had to thoughts. The symptoms of depression in remission are by definition 'low level' and the MBCT course was
designed as a practice-based training that would enable participants to identify
early signs of depression in order to prevent relapse and actively to maintain
their mental health. MBCT participants are encouraged to develop awareness

of small fluctuations in mood, thoughts or bodily experiences. They learn that developing awareness in this way, when the rumblings of depressive symptoms are relatively 'quiet', has the potential to prevent them slipping back into depression.

In what follows, I consider three different modes of learning in MBCT: cognitive, metacognitive and attitudinal. Through ongoing practice-based training, MBCT participants learn to establish a 'friendly' relationship with their own minds in order to prevent depressive relapse. They learn a cognitive theory of mind to account for the experience of depression, and they develop a reflective relationship with their thoughts, feelings and bodily sensations that is characterised by an attitude of 'friendly curiosity'. It is thought that cultivating a 'decentred perspective' or a 'different place to stand' in relation to depressive thoughts is centrally important in the prevention of depressive relapse. Over the eight-week course, participants learn that they *can* develop a relationship with their own minds, and they learn to think of this ability as an important support for their mental health.

In developing this analysis, I seek to challenge the distinction between 'cultural' and 'psychological' approaches to depression. I highlight the historic separation between anthropological attention to culture and psychology's focus on mental processes (see Bruner 1999) and draw ethnographic attention to the mutual construction of mental and social processes. In so doing, I seek to contribute to a growing body of scholarship that examines the interrelationship of culture and mind. Anthropologists and culturally oriented psychologists have shown that mental health is culturally shaped (see, e.g., Cassaniti and Menon 2017; Luhrmann and Marrow 2016; Watters 2010; Wilkinson and Kleinman 2016) revealing the 'similarities and meaningful variations in the psychological experience of illness across cultures' (Horton 2017, 240). An ethnographic focus on MBCT highlights the fact that people who have previously been diagnosed with depression but who are currently well attend to their own mental health through dedicated training in order to prevent depressive relapse and cultivate mental health. Following Hacking (1999, 32), I argue that diagnostic classifications are 'interactive': ways of classifying people interact with those who are so classified. In this context, depression is referred to as a clinical disorder, and mental health is understood as something that can be supported through practices of self-cultivation. I argue that 'psychological' and 'cultural' practices are braided together in changing nosologies of depression and therapeutic intervention. This 'both/and' analysis enables us to think beyond critiques premised on an opposition between categories, and enables us to account for the meaning of depression in a changing landscape of mental health.

Cognition, Metacognition
and a David Attenborough Attitude

I conducted anthropological research at one of the centres in the UK where MBCT is researched, therapists are taught and patients attend courses. The mission of the centre is to improve understanding and treatment of the full 'spectrum' of mood disorders, including major depression and bipolar depression. Under its auspices, research is conducted into psychological therapies and into the psychological processes that underlie the development and maintenance of mood disorders. The centre also aims to improve access to best evidence, research findings and therapies. An adjunct of the centre offers training and continuing practitioner development for health professionals. Clinical work, including the implementation of psychological therapies, occurs at an on-site clinic, which works to develop, test and make accessible effective treatments for depression and other mood disorders. Funded by an NHS Clinical Commissioning Group (CCG), the clinic is housed in a beautiful purpose-built clinical space, which is designed on wending curves and soft lines, with a green living roof. It serves most of the county, working with GP practices and other NHS services including the Depression and Anxiety Service and Mental Wellbeing and Access Teams, providing evidence-based psychological therapies to people in the community who experience severe or recurrent mood disorders. People who wish to participate in an MBCT course at the clinic must be referred via the Depression and Anxiety services, their GP or the local Mental Health Assessment Teams.

MBCT is taught in groups of eight to twelve people, led by a trained therapist, who meet once a week for two hours and fifteen minutes over an eight-week period. The course I refer to in this chapter was held in a large, low-ceilinged room in the clinic. French windows took up one wall of the room and usually looked out onto fine rain falling in a courtyard. We were twelve people, all white and evenly split between men and women. The majority were in their late forties and fifties, two were in their thirties, one was in her twenties, and one was in her late sixties.

Each session of an MBCT course is highly routinised and is made up of mindfulness practices, cognitive exercises and enquiry sessions for discussion. Throughout the week participants are asked to do 'homework': guided mindfulness practices to be completed each day, and exercises such as bringing mindful awareness to specified routine activities and writing pleasant and unpleasant events calendars; in the penultimate week participants also complete a relapse signature chart (charting the signs of their personal relapse into depression) and action plan. Describing her first impressions of the MBCT course in interview, Becky told me that she had felt comforted that everyone was there for the same reason and that they all looked more or less 'normal', as she put it. She had tried a depression support group before beginning MBCT and she had found listening to people's experiences of depression dangerously sad. In the MBCT sessions, discussion focused on the mindfulness techniques and Becky told me that it was helpful to her that the sessions were not 'therapising' depression. Instead, hearing that other people were struggling with the mindfulness practices each week made her feel like she was not alone.

MBCT was developed as a practice-based therapy which enables practitioners to step out of automatic ruminative thinking patterns. The focus of the therapy is not on changing the content of negative thinking but rather is focused on developing the capacity to witness thoughts from a decentred perspective and thereby reduce the authority they have over perceptions of reality. This requires dedicated training on the part of the practitioner. In the cognitive theory of depressive relapse, it is thought that during a depressive episode an association is made between lowered mood and patterns of negative thinking. Once an acute depressive episode has passed, a low mood may trigger automatic patterns of negative thinking, which then reinforce the experience of low mood.

One automatic cognitive strategy for addressing low mood is to ruminate about it in an effort to find a solution and thereby feel better. This ruminative response trait is in the service of solving, or learning about, the 'problem': 'if I could only figure out what was wrong with me . . .'. But the problem-solving thinking employed to find a solution to depression is itself conditioned by a depressogenic schema, and leads to further lowered mood rather than resolution. Self-critical or negative thinking patterns are understood to be habitual and automatic (the person does not 'intend' to be self-critical or negatively judgemental) and in the company of lowered mood, may appear to be accurate reflections on personal inadequacy or failure, which may in turn legitimise and prolong the experience of lowered mood (see Teasdale, Segal and Williams 1995). Thus the perpetuation of negative thoughts about the self will be automatic and highly persuasive.[4] In this cognitive framework, relapse into depression involves a shift of multiple factors in concert: mood lowers, and different thinking patterns begin; at the same time, bodily sensations, behaviour, memory and perception change. Lowered or heightened mood biases interpretations of experience, the ability to recall past events and expectations about the future. Depressed people might recall more negative memories, not only because negative things have happened to them, but also because the negative mood of depression generates negative biases that colour memory, making it easier to recall unpleasant memories and to interpret experience negatively.[5] Thus thoughts, feelings and physical sensations create feedback loops that reinforce each other in a negative spiral, which, if left unchecked, may lead to a depressive relapse.

Through formal practices in class and at home, MBCT participants train metacognitive awareness of negative thoughts and feelings. This is referred to as 'decentring' or 'finding a different place to stand' in order to 'witness' self-criticism, rumination or physical or emotional discomfort. This capacity is epitomised in the refrain used frequently as a shorthand encouragement for cognitive decentring: 'thoughts are not facts'. Metaphors to describe this over the course of the eight weeks include watching clouds that come and go in a blue sky (thoughts make up the weather pattern but they are not the sky), and watching a film or a play (thoughts are like the actors who enter and exit the scene). The development of a decentred perspective from which to view thoughts, feelings and bodily responses is a primary task of mindfulness training, through which participants are learning to 'step aside', to 'shift gear' to a different way of relating to internal and external states. Through meditation practices (for example, by meditating on the breath) participants learn that it is possible to cultivate a witnessing perspective from which to view thoughts and feelings as they arise and pass away, and that this involves relating differently to their experiences. This is also taught through in-class exercises that are intended to illustrate the link between the interpretation of events and moods for participants, and to provide them with an understanding of why it is important to identify thoughts and moods and to be vigilant for the beginning of ruminative thinking. For example, in week two of the course, participants practise an exercise called 'walking down the street', focused on the relationship between thoughts and feelings. In Becky's course, participants were asked to settle into a comfortable seated position. Most people remained in chairs, but some chose to sit on the floor and there was a brief pause as three people fetched cushions from the cupboard in the corner. Once everyone was settled, the therapist, Jane, a smiley woman in her early fifties, asked the group to close their eyes and imagine a scenario:

> You are walking down the street . . . and on the other side of the street you see somebody you know a little way away. . . . You smile and wave at them. . . . The person carries on walking. . . . How do you feel? . . . What thoughts come up in your mind? Do you have any feelings in your body?

Everyone opened their eyes and Jane drew a circle on a flipchart with the word 'situation' around it and two stick figures on either side. She asked the group, 'Would anyone like to start?' Everyone in turn reported a different experience, listing a thought and an accompanying feeling. One woman struggled to decide whom she was 'seeing' and felt that this impacted on her experience of the exercise. Another said, 'I knew exactly who it was!' The therapist prompted each person to delineate distinct thoughts, emotions and bodily sensations. One woman responded, 'Well, I know exactly how I feel in that situation. It's mortifying! I am so embarrassed.' 'What thought did you have?' asked our therapist. 'What feeling came with that? Did any bodily sensations accompany that?' 'Well, embarrassed, I guess,' said the woman. 'And "I'm such a fool," I suppose. My cheeks flush and I can feel my scalp. I can feel it now.' The therapist wrote up 'I'm a fool', 'embarrassment' and 'flushed'.

Another woman said, 'Nothing. I thought that she probably didn't see me so I suppose I carried on down the street.' 'You're shrugging as you say that,' commented our therapist. 'Yes, I suppose I am. So, "easy", I suppose,' the woman responded, shrugging again. 'Didn't see me', 'easy' and 'shrugging' went up on the chart.

Becky interjected as this woman was finishing: 'I was worried that I'd upset him, just "What have I done?" And I felt suddenly flat, like all of the energy had gone out of my chest, like a balloon. So, "worry", I guess.' Each time, the therapist wrote up the thought, feeling, and sensation in the space around the circle until everyone had spoken and the responses filled much of the paper.

This exercise is intended to highlight the fact that a neutral experience can elicit very different interpretations, and that experiences of even a simple exercise may be impactful. Jane used participants' responses to the exercise to teach the group that patterns of interpretation and reaction are a shared part of what it is to be human, and that the 'meaning' of an event has as much to do with the interpretation of it as the event itself. The exercise is also intended to illustrate that lowered mood is strongly correlated with negative interpretations: a negative mood may lead to a negative thought and vice versa; thus, emotional experiences may be determined by thoughts, and thoughts by emotional experiences. Jane told the group that recognising their thoughts and responding skilfully to them is easier if it is done early, because thoughts can provide an interpretation before one is aware that it has happened. 'The challenge', she said, 'is to spot "story making" early enough, because it occurs automatically, and can sweep us away before we realise it's happening.'

One of the primary methods for 'decentring' is awareness of the body, developed through formal and informal practice. The first exercise in which this is learnt is a 'body scan' in which practitioners are guided sequentially to focus attention on different body parts. Participants either lie down or sit comfortably for the exercise and the therapist guides them to focus on different parts of the body in turn. Training to focus attention in this way is intended to develop attentional control and decentring capacity. Participants learn to develop awareness of the body and to engage with physical sensation in new ways. They practise manipulating their focus in order to develop the ability to move it at will. In guided instructions, awareness is described as a 'spotlight' or an 'aperture' which may be narrowed or widened, and the body is described as an 'anchor' for awareness. The therapist guides participants to bring awareness to the physical sensations in each part of the body.[6] Training to focus attention on different parts of the body at will is both an attention training exercise and provides a focus for awareness that is separate from ruminative thinking. By learning to focus awareness in the body, participants are learning to 'decentre' from thinking patterns. At the same time, the participant is learning to be attentive to subtle somatic changes that accompany negative emotions or thoughts. Participants learn to develop awareness of how unpleasant emotion feels in the body—for example, a constriction in the chest, clenching the jaw, or muscular fatigue. Awareness of the body enables the practitioner to recognise bodily experiences, and then choose whether and how to respond to them.

Once the participant is able to hold a particular thought, feeling or bodily sensation in awareness she is encouraged to relate to it in an accepting and kindly way. As one mindfulness teacher put it, participants are learning to relate to themselves with a 'David Attenborough attitude'.[7] 'How do we have an attitude', he said to me, 'that's more friendly, more interested: more like David Attenborough with gorillas than like a sniper with a target?' Participants learn to cultivate attentional control and metacognitive awareness conditioned by an attitude of 'friendly curiosity'. This attitude is not the explicit focus of any formal practices, but instead is intended to infuse the relationship that the practitioner develops with herself. The content of thoughts may or may not be 'friendly', but the participant learns to relate to those thoughts with a mind that is conditioned by compassion. Throughout the course, the therapist's language is welcoming and laced with invitational phrases ('as best you can', 'if it feels comfortable for you') and encourages participants to relate to themselves in kindly ways ('turning towards', 'gently escorting the attention back to the breath', 'softening towards', 'congratulating yourself', 'accepting what is'). Through mindfulness practices and enquiry sessions, participants are encouraged to develop awareness of painful states and to relate to them with kindness, acceptance and patience. They are encouraged to 'soften and open' to experiences. The symptoms of anxiety or depression, such as negative self-judgement, are thereby reframed as depersonalised phenomena and related to with compassion. Practitioners engage in the metacognitive work of learning to experience thought processes *as* thought processes, and they learn to do this with an attitude of compassion and curiosity. That is, the emphasis on 'friendly curiosity' is not in practice an injunction to think particularly happy, loving thoughts. Instead, it is training in relating to thoughts, feelings and emotional states with a friendly 'attitude'. It is this attitudinal disposition, rather than the content of thoughts themselves (which, the practitioner learns, are not facts), that informs metacognitive awareness of thoughts.

The Optimism of Metacognition and Mental Health

As with maintenance antidepressant medication (m-ADMs), MBCT was developed as an intervention for people who are not depressed, but who are statistically likely to experience depressive relapse. MBCT participants learn the cognitive framework for depressive relapse. Through dedicated practice they learn to experience 'thoughts as thoughts' in the progressive development of a relationship with their own minds and the cultivation of a decentred perspective from which to view cognitive, emotional and bodily processes. Formal and informal mindfulness practices are techniques for practitioners to develop attentional control, decentring and 'friendly curiosity'. Thus, MBCT rests on the premise both that there is a cognitive component to depression and that people can learn ways of relating to their thoughts and feelings that can prevent relapse and support mental health.

In his work relating to Inner Mongolia, Jonathan Mair (2013; 2018) has argued that differences in metacognition may lead to dramatically different ways of engaging with knowledge. Focusing on the ways in which Buddhists relate to beliefs, Mair notes (2013, 448) that 'believers are often engaged in complex, reflexive practices that stipulate specific cognitive and non-cognitive relationships to propositional content'. He argues (2018) that focusing on metacognition enables anthropologists to account for the ways in which people reflect on and attempt to act on their own cognition and cognitive experience. For example, the Buddhists with whom Mair works cultivate humility as an appropriate disposition towards the deeper truths of Buddhism. As such, metacognition serves to make the functions of cognition the object of 'self-conscious reflection, ethical evaluation and concerted attempts to mould them into specific forms by building habits, directing attention, associating cognitive functions with emotion and so on' (2018, 412). Comparatively, in the structured learning process of the MBCT course we see a culturally specific valorisation of metacognitive awareness. Metacognition is interpreted as a pan-human ability which can be trained in the prevention of depression and the cultivation of mental health. The MBCT participant does not seek to change her thoughts (for example from depressed to happy), but seeks to develop a relationship towards them (whatever they may be) that is friendly. Thus, in MBCT, metacognitive awareness is explicitly valued as a means by which people might relate to their own objectified minds in the pursuit of living well.

In comparison to alternative framings of depressive relapse, this presents an optimistic picture of mental health. For example, Dumit argues (2002) that in America the reframing of depression from an acute to a recurring or relapsing condition has led to a shift from understanding people as 'inherently healthy' (most people are healthy and most illnesses are temporary interruptions in otherwise healthy lives) to 'inherently ill'. In combination with a theory of genetic causation, framing depression as a relapsing condition rendered people 'only precariously in the "normal state"' (2002, 127), and this had important implications for how people engaged with medication. The new normalcy for people vulnerable to depressive relapse was dependency on medication, evoking what Dumit refers to as a 'pharmaceutical self': 'an individual whose everyday experience of his symptoms is as if he is on bad drugs, too little serotonin perhaps, and in need of good drugs, like an SSRI, to balance the bad one out and bring both biochemistry and symptoms to proper levels' (ibid., 126).[8] The emphasis on awareness training in MBCT suggests a far more optimistic interpretation of the prevention of relapse, one in which the emphasis is placed on the maintenance of mental health through metacognitive training. At the time of engaging with MBCT, participants are well; that is to say, they are not expected to be exhibiting depressive symptoms, but they are understood to be at risk of relapse. Supporting mental health is understood as an ongoing practice that both prevents depression and contributes to health. A shift from 'inherent health' to 'inherent illness', which provided Dumit with a rich analytical framework for understanding genetic interpretations of depressive relapse, thus differs significantly from cognitive interpretations, which emphasise training, cultivation and health.

This is highlighted in week four of the eight-week MBCT course, focused on 'turning towards difficulty' and the types of thoughts that are specifically associated with depression. In the group, each participant received a handout of the Automatic Thoughts Questionnaire (Hollon and Kendall 1980), which comprises of a list of negative self-statements such as 'I'm no good', 'My life is not going the way I want it to', 'I'm worthless', 'My future is bleak', 'I can't finish anything'. The therapist asked them if they recognised any of these statements. 'Some,' said one lady, shifting in her seat, 'Not now, but before . . . yeah, most of them.' There was a palpable drop in the emotional register in the room. One by one participants moved through the list, recognising thoughts that they had had about themselves when they were depressed. Jane encouraged the group to see that these automatic negative thoughts are a symptom of depression rather than 'true'. 'So,' she began, 'we can learn to recognise them. And we can do it again and again. It's like recognising what's on the soundtrack of the mind. And we can find a different place to stand.'

Jane had stuck a laminated poster on the wall, which was slightly tatty around the edges. It had obviously been used in multiple courses and refused to stay blu-tacked at the bottom, curling up at one corner. It showed an image of a figure paddling towards a large waterfall, with the words 'Niagara Falls' printed above it. Jane pointed to the picture to describe the effects of negative thinking:

> Once negative thinking starts it may be hard to stop. It's a bit like being pulled towards the falls and no matter how hard we paddle, we're not strong enough to stop ourselves being pulled over. We're far up stream, and it's a beautiful day, we can hear the noise of the falls in the distance but it's far away and we're not really paying attention. Then before we know it, we are moving faster and faster and so we start paddling as hard as we can, but no matter what we do, we can't stop ourselves. We're being sucked over, again.

The spectre of depression loomed up around our circle as she spoke, and the world narrowed. I felt, weakly, that we had been building a sense of shared endeavour, and that the inevitability of depression had been lurking in the

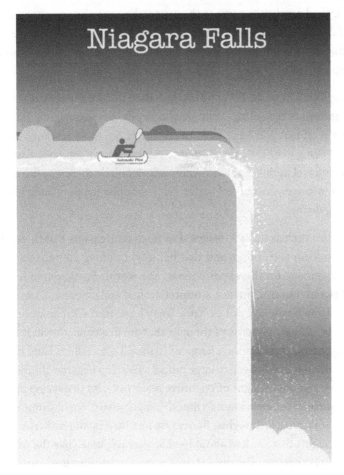

FIGURE 2. The image of Niagara Falls used in the MBCT
course, as published in Feldman and Kuyken (2011).

background the whole time. 'But by paying attention,' Jane went on, 'we can
begin to learn the early signs of negative thinking before they get too loud, and
we can find a different place to stand.' This, she told us,

> is mindfulness. We're learning to notice. Notice the small movements. We can
> notice that our thinking is becoming negative and we can step to one side.
> When we feel the current quicken, and hear the falls in the distance, why not
> paddle to the bank and carry that canoe for a little bit? We don't have to be
> dragged down every thinking spiral. By noticing it when it's quiet we have
> a choice about what we do, before it gets too loud and it's too hard.

Becky had nearly not come to the session because she was struggling. She arrived desolate, feeling both depressed and furious with herself for feeling so low while she was on the course. But the focus on turning toward difficulty, to her surprise, led to an epiphany. She told me afterwards,

> It was like, 'Oh, yeah.' If I'm feeling low, then just accepting that I'm feeling low instead of being like, 'Why are you *bloody well* feeling low?' It's a whole other level that you don't need to engage in. So, there is something there about being like, 'OK, stop trying to . . . this is how you feel . . . and that's how you feel in this moment.' And yeah, definitely there's stuff you can do to try to make yourself feel better, but it stopped me punishing myself for feeling down.

Exercises such as this are designed to teach participants that thoughts and feelings inform each other, and that habitual thinking patterns can exert a strong influence on the experience of the world. Participants learn that thoughts and moods influence interpretation of and reaction to experiences, and that thoughts might not be 'true'. They learn that a dip in mood has the potential to trigger patterns of thought that are disproportionately negative and judgemental ('This always happens to me'; 'I am a failure') and that small changes in mood might lead to large modal shifts into negative thinking. They learn to be vigilant for signs of 'cognitive reactivity' and to develop awareness of a relationship between lowered mood and negative thought patterns. As she began to observe her thoughts, Becky was horrified by the realisation that all of the thoughts that she had about herself were negative, 'like the *whole* time everything is negative, everything I do is wrong, everything is wrong'. Towards the end of the course participants are asked to complete a relapse signature chart, listing how they feel and behave as their mood lowers in order that they might prepare a skilful response for each stage. Becky began to see many of the things that she had been blaming herself for as symptoms of depression. As she told me, 'I was just like, "Oh!" I thought that was just me being really bad at being a grown-up, but no, that's actually being depressed.'

After her course, Becky told me that she started to feel relief from her brutal self-criticism as she began to depersonalise negative thoughts and understand them instead as the symptoms of depression. She aspired to develop 'friendly curiosity' towards herself but, she told me, 'It's still a challenge. Both the friendliness and the curiosity.' But she could muster 'acceptance', which she thought was pretty good going, really. Becky describes her thoughts when she is depressed as 'sneaky voices': 'They're sneaky because they sound like they're trying to help,' she says. 'In the past if I was hearing really negative voices or feeling very low, I wouldn't be able to see beyond it. I'd think the voices were real, and that the feelings were absolute.' Now she relates differently to her thoughts and recognises the impulse to take herself into isolation as a symptom of depression:

> To hear the voices and be like, 'Yep, there it is.' But it's not real. And the same in my mood, again being aware of it as something that's changing. I'll still have times when I feel terrible, but I know that they're not going to last forever and I'm much more aware of what I can do to make myself feel better.

Becky monitors her thoughts and behaviour for patterns that might precipitate descent back into depression, and she has a clear sense of what kinds of behaviour may be symptomatic of depression (ignoring mail and email, isolating herself from others) and what kinds of activities are helpful for maintaining her health (for Becky, being with others, exercise and meditation). Staying well for Becky involves understanding both what triggers a lowered mood and how she can support herself when things are hard.

The 'Culture' and 'Psychology' of Depression

Depression poses a challenge to social scientific analysis. Much of the earlier work of the interpretivists and culture and personality theorists rested on an interest in psychological variation and interior subjectivity, and the degree to which these varied cross-culturally.[9] What each of these scholars argued, in diverse ways, is that human experience cannot be compressed into the categories of modern psychiatry and psychology, and to attempt so to compress it denatures understanding of people's suffering (see Brown 1995). This scholarship highlighted the possibility that depression may be an expression of socially produced demoralisation and that psychiatric formulations may not be sufficient to account for expressions of depression-like experience (see also Kleinman 1986; 1988; Kleinman and Good 1985).[10] Alternatively, some have suggested that the prevalence of depression is the result of successful marketing campaigns that have expanded the diagnosis to fuel the sale of antidepressants (see Healy 1997). Critics have argued that therapy goes too far in medicalising everyday depression: changes in diagnostic criteria, which do not contextualise symptoms, have led to the misclassification of normal emotional responses to sadness as mental disorder (Horwitz and Wakefield 2007). Thus, the rise in the global prevalence of depression is taken as an example of the ways in which the problems of living come to be reinterpreted as issues of individual psychology. Some have developed this further to argue that psychological reductionism may lead to surveillance (Lupton 1997), depoliticisation (Young 1995) and control (see Rose 2007).[11]

Is depression a disorder? A dimension of the human condition? A culturally specific category? An appropriate response to circumstantial or structural realities? 'Depression' can signify all of these things. In common usage, it can refer to a transitory mood or emotion that is experienced by everyone, a discrete form of pathology, a diagnosis of a psychiatric disorder, a symptom of a mental disorder (such as anxiety disorder, or schizophrenia) or a symptom of other diseases (such as cardiovascular disease, post-viral syndromes or thyroid disorders). And this slippage of meanings risks conflating everyday emotional experience with pathological suffering. Social, political and economic factors have repeatedly been demonstrated to contribute to the diagnosis and prevalence of major depression and human suffering more broadly (see, e.g., Adler et al. 1994). Low socioeconomic status, unstable home environments and lack of social connectedness have all been shown to impact mental health (WHO 2012; see also NICE 2009). For example, in England, prescriptions for antidepressants increased from fifteen million in 1996 to forty million in 2012, and over half of this increase occurred in the four years following the 2008 financial crisis (Spence et al. 2014). Spence et al. hypothesise that contributing factors to this increase were the growth in unemployment, poverty and inequality caused by the economic recession, leading to increasing mental health problems and demand for health services.

At the same time, depression is not *only* an economic or structural problem. Major depression is not limited to mood; it affects a person's ability to think clearly, to sleep, to eat. It is recognised as a factor contributing to addiction, suicide, difficult relationships, self-diminishment and much barefaced misery. Feelings of isolation, worthlessness, despair, unbearable mental pain and suffering characterise the disorder. Acutely depressed people cannot concentrate. They may have trouble communicating and lack the motivation to leave their beds.[12] People who suffer from depression may be obsessed with thoughts of their own death, and the risk of suicide increases with each new episode.[13] Even the most articulate of those who have suffered from depression, among them Emily Dickinson, John Donne and Virginia Woolf, have struggled to find words for their experience. William James, who battled with depression for much of his life, wrote of this impossibility, 'It is positive and active anguish, a sort of psychical neuralgia wholly unknown to normal life' (James 2020 [1902], 83). William Styron likened it (1990) to drowning or suffocation, but still felt this was a poor representation. In a fiction that mirrored her life, Sylvia Plath wrote (1966, 278), 'To the person in the bell jar, blank and stopped as a dead baby, the world itself is a bad dream'.[14] Participants who have completed an MBCT course described their earlier experiences of depression to me in similarly opaque terms. Some described a gradual numbing, as life becomes less colourful, mornings more sluggish. Others told me about insistent spikes of anxiety, peaking ever higher. Everyone spoke of transformations in speech, movement and social interaction, and transformed experiences of their bodies: bodily twitches and aches plague waking life, a counterpoint to the fidgeting or listlessness brought on by sleeping too much or too little, or total absence of any feeling at all.

In emphasising the cultural construction of distress and diagnosis, scholars were able to examine cross-cultural variance. This, however, as O'Nell argues (1998), disallowed the notion of depression as a universal category. It inhibited the possibility of asking whether an individual or a group of people was 'really' depressed and of examining the degree to which culture masks the presentation of depression. By questioning the psychiatric formulation of depression-like experiences, scholars were thereby 'rendering moot questions about depression as an entity in this cultural setting and focusing instead on locally constructed realities' (1998, 10). For all the critique of psychological categories and diagnoses, none of it comes as much of a surprise. It is reasonably uncontroversial to demonstrate that a medical system, like all social activity, is influenced by demands, risks, politics, power struggles, structural inequalities and so on. What is surprising about such critiques is the implication that they are *only* that (see Stengers 2000, 13). The challenge of some critical approaches is that they imply that the *real* causes of and solutions to depression are structural, not psychological. In so doing, an opposition is established between psychological and cultural influences. One of the challenges of this is that such critiques leave little recourse to address the experiences of those who are currently suffering and who understand themselves to have a diagnosable condition.

For people with depression, the advice about what to do can be baffling, and the urgency with which help is needed can be desperate. Psychological understandings of depression have been transformed by successive theories of causation and therapeutic approaches. There is no doubt that in certain moderate cases of depressive episodes, and some chronic cases, medication can prove invaluable, and that in some cases it can alter the course of a serious episode. In its early stages, depression is said to respond well to techniques such as cognitive therapy and other psychiatric strategies, alone or in combination with medication. But even in frameworks that characterise depressive symptoms as being caused by genetic, cognitive or neurochemical mechanisms, depression remains contingent, subject to social influence, evaluation and contestation. Radically different interpretations of the causes of depression, reflected in ongoing tensions between psychotherapy and pharmacology, impact the meaning of illness, intervention in response to it, and its alleviation. There are good works of advice that thoughtfully explain appropriate possible interventions and treatments, clarifying how different therapies, such as psychotherapy or pharmacology, or a combination of approaches, might help to restore and maintain health; but most good advice highlights the fact that alleviating serious depression takes time, and it is not always clear how best to address it.

One way of bridging the gap between anthropological and psychological approaches to diagnostic categories might be pragmatic: while the categorisation of depressive disorders as disease-specific certainly represents a reductionist account of human suffering (how could it not?), it may be a sufficient and necessary classification in order to enable practical decision-making about treatment (see Kirmayer 1991). In such an approach, diagnostic categories act as heuristics: utilitarian or reductionist ways of getting stuff done in a complicated world. The disease-specificity model might be interpreted as a reductionist means to achieve necessarily holistic ends, in culturally appropriate terms, in order to attend to the needs of suffering individuals. This tension between 'cultural' and 'psychological' approaches to depression is one that Teresa O'Nell addresses in her ethnography of loneliness among the Flathead native group in North America. Flathead reports of depressive experience are characterised by social responsibility and familial respect, both of which are understood as signs of maturity and Native American identity (1998, 7).[15] O'Nell argues that accounting for depression through the different but important perspectives of psychiatry and anthropology requires analytically oscillating between two different vantage points, one characterised by distanced overview and the other by ensconced meaning. In the metaphor she uses, the researcher must 'be capable of running back and forth between Main Street and the spot across the bridge' (ibid., 210).

In this chapter I have sought to provide a 'both/and' alternative to the analytic distinction between 'psychological' and 'cultural' knowledge. Therapeutic interventions for the prevention of depressive relapse are premised on the idea that people who have recovered from acute depression maintain a latent vulnerability to relapse. In addition to this rethinking of the classification of depression, those whose conditions are so classified may behave differently, for example, by participating in a therapeutic intervention for the prevention of relapse. People who participate in MBCT programmes are taught, through cognitive, metacognitive and attitudinal training, to think about and relate to their experience in new ways and this change informs their experience and understanding of depression. I refer to this as a 'both/and' analysis because depression is understood both as a clinical diagnosis and as something that can be addressed through ongoing training. Thus this analysis of mental health and health-seeking behaviour does not pit psychological and cultural causation or constitution against each other in a zero-sum relationship. This moves us from an analysis of the veracity of diagnostic categories to an ethnographic focus on the cultivation of a culturally specific understanding of mental health, reframing previously discrete alternatives of diagnostic categories and situated human experience as interwoven in interactive relationships, rather than as discrete alternatives.[16] As others have noted, dialogue across the historical disciplinary divide between anthropology and psychology contributes to the emergence of culturally hybrid forms of mental healthcare (see Kirmayer 2006) and highlights the ways in which experiences of mental illness and healthcare are affected by beliefs and expectations embedded in culture (see Cassaniti and Menon 2017; Watters 2010).[17]

As the foregoing representation indicates, diverse social scientific critiques of psychiatric authority and diagnostic epistemology have provided a spirited and multivocal analysis of depression. However, far from doing away with the psychological categories or discourses of mental health, five decades of critique have contributed to contemporary understandings in which, paradoxically, a 'fundamental scepticism coexists with a triumphalist reductionism' (Rosenberg 2015, 131). Lexicons of disease categories are both nurtured and contested, even as they expand, and as critical sentiment is incorporated into contemporary understandings of health. As Hacking notes (1999), the classification of people into categories is unlike other forms of classification, because people are aware of what is thought about them and this informs the ways in which they think about and conceptualise themselves. For example, people who are given a diagnosis of depression become aware that they are classified in such a way: '[t]hey can make tacit or even explicit choices, adapt or adopt ways of living so as to fit or get away from the very classification that may be applied to them. These very choices, adaptations, or adoptions have consequences for the very group, for the kind of people that is invoked' (Hacking 1999, 34; see also Hacking 1995a). Hacking refers to this as 'the looping effect of human kinds': people are classified as particular kinds, and because kinds can interact with what is classified, the classification may be modified or replaced. In this way, 'psychological' and 'cultural' forms of knowledge are interactive.

In this 'both/and' analysis of MBCT I have sought to account for contemporary British framings of mental health as amenable to psychosocial support. The shift from treating depression in an acute state to an emphasis on preventative interventions, such as MBCT, is part of broader changes in the way that people understand mental health in Britain. As we will see in the next chapter, mental health is increasingly thought of as 'something we all have' and something that can be actively supported. This is informed by optimistic ideas about the human mind and the potential of psychological knowledge and practices to support living well. For mindfulness practitioners, metacognitive awareness is understood to be a universal human capacity that may be cultivated. The view underpinning this understanding is that everyone would benefit from developing a decentred and healthy relationship with themselves by practising mindfulness. As we have seen, MBCT participants cultivate an active orientation towards their own minds by developing a relationship between metacognitive training, cognitive knowledge and attitudinal disposition in order to prevent depressive relapse and cultivate mental health. The aim of this is to develop a kindly relationship with the mind through attentional control, and the strategies for developing these abilities are formal and informal mindfulness practices. My ethnographic examination of depression and mental healthcare for MBCT participants reflects the ongoing relationship between diagnostic categories, meaning and experience.

3

Mindfulness in the Extraordinary Ordinary

Beauty, the world seemed to say. And as if to prove it (scientifically) wherever he looked at the houses, at the railings, at the antelopes stretching over the palings, beauty sprang instantly. To watch a leaf quivering in the rush of air was an exquisite joy.

—VIRGINIA WOOLF, MRS DALLOWAY

IN VIRGINIA WOOLF'S *Mrs Dalloway* (1925), the two central characters experience moments of intense awareness of what appear to be trivial particularities. Clarissa Dalloway finds passing taxis 'absolutely absorbing' and she closes her eyes to take in the full scent of the flowers in Miss Pym's shop; Septimus Warren Smith is exalted by the rising and falling of elm trees in Regent's Park, 'with all their leaves alight and the colour thinning and thickening from blue to the green of a hollow wave'. The temporal arc of *Mrs Dalloway* spans a few hours in an ordinary day, a period during which, according to literary standards, very little usually happens. But the day that Clarissa Dalloway lives is significant for its sheer everydayness and Woolf emphasises her characters' acute consciousness of ordinary moments. In a collection of autobiographical essays published after her death (Woolf 1985), Woolf characterises such experiences as 'moments of being', and she wonders why some moments are so powerful, even if the events contained within them are themselves unimportant, while others are easily forgotten. For Woolf, what separates moments of 'being' from moments of 'non-being' is consciousness of the experiences that they contain. One act is no more extraordinary or mundane than another. Routine activities (she specifies walking and shopping) are moments of

non-being when they are carried out unthinkingly, embedded in 'a kind
of nondescript cotton wool' (1985, 70) and it is consciousness of experience
that separates these from moments of being, which are experienced with intensity and awareness.

I begin this chapter with Woolf's moments of being in order to point to the
'everydayness' of mindfulness in 'ordinary' life for dedicated practitioners.
Over the course of two years' participant observation with mindfulness therapists in training, I was puzzled by the contrastive way in which they engaged
with mindfulness in their own lives: practitioners described mindfulness both
as utterly ordinary and as deeply profound. They practised mindful awareness
in the mundane and routine activities of daily life. It was highly quotidian,
aimed not at transcendence but at the experience of being with or being near
emotional and cognitive experience, as practitioners asked themselves if they
could be mindful 'in the midst of' life. But mindfulness was also described as
enabling a quality of engagement with ordinary activities by which practitioners
might live more fully and be more 'awake'. As a result of practice, mundane experiences took on new meaning and were thought of as 'miraculous' and extraordinary. Practitioners sometimes described mindfulness as a way of managing and ameliorating difficult emotional experiences, and at other times as
a profoundly transformative ethical practice, simultaneously a pragmatic technique for responding to daily stress and a radically different 'way of being'.
Mindfulness appeared to be both instrumental and ethical, everyday and
exceptional.

The problem of the basic knowability of the everyday vexes much scholarship on the subject. How might we define 'the everyday'? Is it best understood
in terms of ordinariness, givenness or normalcy, or is it better accounted for in
terms of repetition, seriality or rhythm? Are everyday acts events in the 'here
and now' rather than the long term? Or are they a type of (daily) activity?[1]
Lefebvre asks (1991 [1958], 38), 'Where is [the everyday] to be found? In work
or in leisure? In family life and in moments "lived" outside of culture?', puzzling
over what he thinks of as an 'obscurity' in the concept of 'everyday life' itself.
For Highmore, everyday life is characterised by a quality of 'everydayness', an
'unspecific gravity' in the way that it is experienced. It may be boring and
relentlessly routinised, but it also contains the potential for mystery. As Highmore writes (2002, 1),

the most travelled journey can become the dead weight of boredom, the
most inhabited space a prison, the most repeated action an oppressive

routine. Here the everydayness of everyday life might be experienced as a sanctuary, or it may bewilder or give pleasure, it may delight or depress. Or its special quality might be its lack of qualities. It might be, precisely, the unnoticed, the inconspicuous, the unobtrusive.

But this 'everydayness' presents us with a paradox: the everyday is both ubiquitous and non-special and once we draw attention to it, it is no longer concurrent with life itself (Sheringham 2006; see also Blanchot 1993, 238–9). As Sayeau puts it (2013, 12), the 'everyday' 'is the name we give to what remains unmarked, undifferentiated, ordinary beyond noticing—to notice it is to transform it into something else, something not quite everyday'. Thus, the everyday is difficult to discover, and in the act of discovering it, it disappears. As Sayeau writes (ibid.), in drawing attention to the everyday, '"it" is no longer everyday, but a significant occurrence, a meaningful example, an event. In a tormenting inversion of the *idée reçue* about pornography—that you know it when you see it—we no longer know the everyday once we have seen it, especially once we have said that we have seen it.' The everyday is all around us and yet it is an elusive level of lived experience that is only seen in moments of depreciation, when it weighs too heavily upon us, or in moments when it is glorified into something that usually it is not.

One way of approaching the everyday is through synonyms, such as 'ordinary', 'habitual', 'mundane' or 'routine'; it is 'that which goes without saying', a habituation to the world that rests on tacit understanding. But discussions of 'ordinary life' share the same challenge as those of 'the everyday'. To speak of ordinary life requires that we enquire into its constitution as an ethnographic object in relation to broader social and cultural structures. And in so doing, either we lift the ordinary out of the undifferentiated flow of life, or the analysis of it rests on a tautologous givenness of the category that is intended to be explored (for excellent critiques on this point in Wittgenstein and Ordinary Language Philosophy, see Gellner 1960; Heywood 2022). The problem of studying the 'ordinary' and the 'everyday' is an assumption that they *are* ordinary or everyday—that we know them when we see them—and that is what makes them an appropriate focus of study, creating a challenge that is complicated further by the necessarily subjective nature of ordinary experience. On the one hand, the 'ordinariness' of life must to some extent be in the eye of the beholder. For example, my daily routine of sitting in cafés, writing this book on my laptop, may seem unordinary and exotic to someone who lives, and works, in an entirely different way. Similarly, the lives of other people, while ordinary to them, may seem extraordinary and exciting to me. On the other hand, 'ordinary' activities may no longer be 'everyday' when they are engaged with in a non-ordinary way. It is possible that routine 'everyday' activities have very different meanings for different people, depending on the intention that is brought to them. A focus, analytical or ethnographic, on ordinary experience lifts it out of the undifferentiated flow of life.

In this chapter, I focus on mindfulness practitioners who intentionally pluck mundane activities out of the flow of daily life by bringing mindful awareness to them. I draw on my relationships with mindfulness therapists to think about the ways in which mindfulness is incorporated into everyday life. They describe mindfulness as a daily practice of tending to their minds in order to cultivate metacognitive and kindly awareness of their thoughts, feelings and bodily sensations, and they describe this experience as 'profound'. Part of the ambition of this chapter, then, is to enquire into what happens when cultivating non-ordinary awareness becomes a part of ordinary life. In what follows I will unpack the ways in which practitioners problematise 'ordinary' experience, and why it matters to them that they do so. What do mindfulness practitioners mean, when they say that unreflective everyday life leads to mental ill-health? And what do they mean when they say that ordinary life is the site of extraordinary experience? I hope to show that 'ordinary' experience is invested with both positive and negative value by practitioners and that, in the light of this, they develop metacognitive reflection in the course of mundane activities both as an instrumental tool for managing difficult emotions and as an ethical practice for living more 'fully'. This analytic focus on the modalities by which people relate to even the most mundane experiences raises broader questions for anthropology. How is metacognitive awareness integrated into the situated practice of daily life? What place does reflective awareness have for practitioners amidst the competing demands, psychological and circumstantial, of life? And is the everyday still 'everyday' when we pay attention to it?

The Problem and the Potential of Ordinary Experience

Dinah is a counsellor in a secondary school in the south-west of England. She began practising mindfulness because she wanted to be proactive about her mental health. Dinah's mother had had three major episodes of depression over the course of Dinah's life and it scared Dinah that, despite her mother being a positive and vivacious woman, when she was depressed, she was powerless to do anything about it: her mother 'very much felt when she was depressed that that was how it was and I don't think she was able to take any active part in that, it's just what happened to her. So that motivated me to think that I can do something to help myself in this.' Never having had depression herself, Dinah signed up for an eight-week mindfulness course in 2012, but the content of the first session left her stumped:

> I remember thinking, 'My god, there's a lot of sitting still and being quiet.' Thinking, 'I don't quite know what this is.' And looking back there was very much this expectation of the hungry bird waiting to be fed—'What are you going to give me?'—and nothing really came.

At home after the first session she told her two children that she would be using the sitting room for meditation and that they were to stay upstairs. She had just lain down on the carpet and closed her eyes to begin the body scan when her ten-year-old son charged into the room:

> I can still remember how my body was, I can't tell you, I was absolutely furious, and it took over my body and I didn't know what to do with it. Reaction is an understatement. I was *furious*. I settled into it and the whole way through the body scan, I sobbed my heart out, the whole way through, because I could feel that I was allowing myself to give in to it. And all the contraction fell away and I just sobbed.

I asked Dinah to tell me what had been 'contracted' as she began the practice, and she pointed to a broad struggle over a long period:

> It was around trying and forcing and wanting things to be a certain way. About trying to control everything in my life. It had been quite a difficult decade in terms of marriage breakdown and problems with my son and everything, and just trying to keep all those plates spinning but doing it in a way where I was very harsh on myself. And not allowing things to be— just getting completely caught up in the striving of it all. It was ruling me at the time.

But, she added, 'There was something quite nice about the sobbing.'

Dinah's first experiences of meditation revealed strong emotions and uncomfortable feelings, associated with larger issues of marriage breakdown and challenging children. She thought that these emotions were already there, but it was only when she 'allowed' herself to feel them in meditation that she stopped being 'caught up' in them. As she told me, reflecting on those experiences after four years of practice,

> The value of actually knowing what your relationship with your own mind is, is huge. Lots of people don't have a relationship with their minds. They live on autopilot. They don't even know that they can think and do things that they're not aware of. And when you're in difficulty and struggling, you're incapacitated completely, and what does that lead to? It leads to shit feeling, acting out, and feeling out of control. It's quite simple when you put it like that. Let's just know our minds, let's know the inclinations, the territory of our minds.

For Dinah, initial experiences of mindfulness practice are figured against what she now thinks of as the psychological costs of being unaware of difficult emotional experiences. In her opinion, part of the challenge of everyday life is the mode in which it is experienced: people are understood to be on 'autopilot' most of the time, habitually engaging in activities while the mind is on other things, which contributes to feeling out of control. Dinah's post-hoc assessment of herself as disconnected from her emotions reflects a broader concern amongst mindfulness practitioners that the habits of everyday life cut people off from emotional experience and contribute to ill-health. Such concerns rest on a negative critique of ordinary life: isolation, atomisation and ill-health are exacerbated by the mode in which the everyday is experienced. The everyday here is associated with habit and a lack of awareness, a rhythmic, banal continuity that persists outside of awareness as the psychological mode of 'autopilot' perpetuates suboptimal mental health.

Common among practitioners was a sense that, before they learned to meditate, they had had a limited awareness of their emotional habits. Susan, brought up as a Quaker, had worked in mental health before leaving the NHS to run a guest-house in Cornwall with her husband. Though she had heard of mindfulness before, in 2011 she was listening to the radio when she caught Mark Williams giving an interview about MBCT. As she told me, 'He just led a minute of silence and that was it, that was the moment, that triggered me to find out more about it, to buy his book, and to start practicing.' Susan says of herself that at the time when she began to practise, 'I couldn't slow down, I was busy all the time and I realised I was making myself busy to not be in touch with myself, with my emotions, thoughts. I was just running from myself without knowing.' Her reflection that she was 'running from herself' echoes a broader suspicion that in everyday life something important is missing in terms of the individual's relationship to society. A common concern in popular commentary about mental health is that modern life is leading to forms of mental ill-health, that people have become alienated from their 'true' selves, and that connection with others too has been lost. For example, Jon Kabat-Zinn writes of America (2005, 146), 'It is now harder to pay attention to any one thing and there is more to pay attention to. [. . .] Things come at us fast and furious, relentlessly. [. . .] These assaults on our nervous system continually stimulate and foster desire and agitation rather than contentedness and calmness.' The everyday emerges as site of critique at a time of heightened anxiety about mental health, and learning to relate differently to everyday activities is thought to ameliorate the disconnection of unreflective modern life. As Susan said to me, 'mental health is not just what you think, it's *how* you think as well'. For Dinah, this propelled her to be proactive about her mental health by trying to develop a relationship with her own mind. 'Mindfulness made me feel active in my own well-being', she told me, 'and it didn't matter where you were on the spectrum, whether you were in the depths of awful things or you were flourishing, you could benefit from it.'

But the everyday is not just the site for a 'realist' or functionalist re-engagement with experience that will help manage emotions or reduce stress. For practitioners, it is also informed by a positive idea of the everyday as the site for flourishing, happiness and wonder. The pragmatism of practices that are intended to enable people to live less stressed-out lives is complemented by a Romantic aspiration to 'live fully' by learning to relate differently to ordinary life. 'Everyday' activities take a central role in mindfulness practice. The historian of religion David McMahan argues (2008, 221) that contemporary adaptations of mindfulness have been informed by 'the distinctively modern valuation of ordinary life as itself the locus of sacrality'. He argues that mindfulness has been inflected with a modernist sensibility in which the details of everyday life are valorised, the ordinary comes to be revered, and in it are discovered universal forms: 'One withdraws from things, or from one's habitual reactions to things, but in such a withdrawal lies the possibility of apprehending a deeper mystery lying within them' (ibid., 234). The practitioners with whom I work think that the normal attitude with which routine or habitual activities are approached is one of 'autopilot'—they occur while the mind is occupied with other things—and that engaging with them in a qualitatively different way leads to a deeper appreciation of experience. In such a view, the quality of engagement that one brings to the circumstances of one's life may provide a locus of meaning and fulfilment. Life is to be lived in the present moment and the everyday is valorised positively. Mark Williams writes, for example, in his popular book *Mindfulness: A Practical Guide to Finding Peace in a Frantic World*, that mindfulness leads to 'the kind of happiness and peace that gets into your bones and promotes a deep-seated authentic love of life, seeping into everything you do and helping you cope more skillfully with the worst that life throws at you' (Williams and Penman 2011, 2; for a discussion of this, see chapter 4 below).

In this sense, everyday life is invested with a positive potential, containing within itself the possibility of its own existential transformation (Sheringham 2006, 12). Practising mindfulness is explicitly associated with an aspiration towards living a life in which one is fully 'present'. The association between 'living a life of presence' and mental health is explicitly stated by Jon Kabat-Zinn when he says (2005, 9) that 'the journey toward health and sanity is nothing less than an invitation to wake up to the fullness of our lives'. Bringing awareness to the present moment, learning to 'be' with what is, without trying to fix or change anything, is described often as bringing a 'freshness' to lived experience, a direct perception of the world. The world comes alive in all of its extraordinary ordinariness, not as a result of any external changes in the world itself, but as a result of the quality of awareness that is brought to perceiving it. Being mindful of mundane activities recasts the 'meaning' of those activities for practitioners. For example, the much-quoted Vietnamese meditation master Thich Nhat Hanh encourages practitioners washing the dishes 'to wash the dishes', that is, to be present with the experience of washing (Nhat Hanh 2008, 4):

> Why put so much stress on a simple thing? But that's precisely the point. The fact that I am standing there and washing these bowls is a wondrous reality. I'm being completely myself, following my breath, conscious of my presence, and conscious of my thoughts and actions.

In this way, mindfulness is brought into the most banal activities of life, such as washing up, and these activities are then approached with an intentionally different attitude. Mindfulness practices in this sense are world-affirming: the good life is to be found within quotidian experience by engaging with it in a particular way (see Taylor 1989, 211–304). The 'miracle of mindfulness', as Nhat Hanh's classic book is titled, is that through world-affirming practice the 'ordinary' is sacralised and made extraordinary.

What marks the everyday as profound is a quality of awareness brought into ordinary activities, and the value of this ongoing practice in everyday life.

Lynn had been a therapist for six years before she began practising mindfulness in 2012, though she had learnt meditation as a *sanyasin* following the teachings of Osho twenty years before. She told me that she thought of this as a 'soft transcendence':

> When you're in the moment, being really present with your washing up or your tea or whatever, it feels like it's a bit transcendent, a soft transcendence maybe. But it's not because you've ascended to somewhere else but because you've really come down into where you are right then.

Leslie, a long-term yoga teacher and Buddhist meditation practitioner, also described mindfulness as profound, but in contrast to Lynn, she didn't think it was transcendent at all. She told me that

> transcendence would just be another way I'd punish myself. Transcendence is a goal, and even though it's not, it kind of is. And so, it's funny, because although there are some really instrumental elements in mindfulness it almost feels less instrumental because I'm not trying to get somewhere. It's about being where I am. And it's about helping me live. It's not about any kind of achieving.

Though they disagree about whether or not mindfulness is transcendent, Lynn's and Leslie's views share a striking conception of both the 'ordinariness' and profundity of daily practice. Lynn and Leslie experience profundity in prosaic activities (washing up, drinking tea) in which very little has actually happened.

This positive valorisation of ordinary experience was emphasised to me by John, a therapist in his fifties. He had joined a Buddhist group when he was younger, but felt frustrated at the degree of faith that was placed in the teacher: 'It rubbed me a little bit,' he told me. 'I was like, "OK, I like the meditation, I like the wisdom." But, having never had any faith before, when someone says, "He's the man!", I question that.' John had a background in outdoor education and had originally heard about mindfulness through a course on group psychology and group dynamics, but he only took it up in earnest after his divorce:

> I was feeling pretty crap about myself and my life at that point. I was then described as 'a divorced man.' It's something I'd never thought I'd be; my parents were together for life. So, there was this change in who I was. I thought, 'Right, I've got to manage myself as this entity'.

John's first eight-week course was run by an art therapist 'in a church, ironically', and then, eighteen months later, his GP referred him to a second course run by two CBT therapists. For John, meditation provided a reappraisal of his relationship with himself by bringing awareness to mundane activities:

> Last week, I was doing a drive somewhere, and I noticed that my mind was flipping in and out of a hundred different things. And then a little voice said, 'What's the quality of your thinking now?', and I thought, 'Crap, actually.' I couldn't pin it down if I tried. And so then I came back to the feeling of the steering wheel, the seat, and then I noticed colours around me, where I was, you know, and everything sort of slowed down and came in. Just through that little question.

For John, this slowing down and coming in is world-affirming and found in routine activities that would normally not be the focus of awareness. He told me that approaching prosaic activities in this way helped him to manage his feelings about his divorce:

> At the time, it was helpful. It gave me structure, it started my practice, but it was only as months went on after that that I found little things, like if I was feeling rubbish or low, I would do my 'drawer cleaning exercise'.

He would clean out and organise the drawers in his kitchen as mindfully as he could,

> because it was really peculiarly helpful. It focused the mind and had that sense of mastery afterwards. And that simplicity and focus I think drew me back to what mindfulness was. That it doesn't have to be grand, deep, euphoric or [that] somehow an epiphany happens during it. None of that. Everyday stuff, everyday moments.

Here, the everyday becomes the site for a re-engagement with life. Daily life is imbued with Epicurean virtues as individual acts (driving, cleaning out drawers) are singled out from the rest of life. Each becomes an individual island of experience, separated from the undifferentiated flow of everyday life. But each act (or 'mindful moment') so reconceived is intended to contribute to a transformed sense of awareness or wakefulness overall. Speaking about running her guest-house, Susan tells me that she finds a bridge between her upbringing as a Quaker and her mindfulness by cleaning and preparing rooms in silence:

> I've noticed now that I hardly ever have the radio on, and I hardly ever watch the television. I mean I know I'm on the iPad all the time, but I love silence. I just love being silent and having silence around me.

She values silence in her day-to-day life as a support for cultivating awareness:

> It's about being focused on what I'm doing. I'm aware that I'm often doing lots of things at once but perhaps I'm being more focused on one thing at a time because of the silence.

There is an interesting comparison to be drawn with other health practices that emphasise positive health. For example, Farquhar and Zhang explore (2012) the contemporary *yangsheng* movement in Beijing, an enthusiasm for life-nurturing theory and practice. Yangsheng actions are characterised by the cultivation of healthy everyday habits. The principles of yangsheng are expressed in 'ordinary everyday life' in efforts to 'harmonise' life in a world made up of 'ten thousand things' (2012, 154). As Farquhar and Zhang's ethnography makes clear, the popularity of yangsheng in contemporary Beijing reflects forms of pleasure and enjoyment that far exceed the utilitarian. As they write (ibid, 130), 'what is cultivated in Beijing's parks and alleyways are not lives of quiet desperation. One hears in so many voices a great emphasis on the pleasures of life nurturance in itself; this testimony must be taken seriously.' For practitioners of yangsheng, health is not the objective of an instrumental technique, but a daily, ongoing practice. Yangsheng advice is almost entirely quotidian, focusing on practical suggestions such as the timing of meals or wearing appropriate clothing, and is often presented as rules of thumb. The philosophy of yangsheng is less about a form of transcendence and more about living on in a state of moderate well-being: 'It advocates a craftwork of the well-formed life, not a quest for the ultimate meanings of life and death' (ibid., 126). As in yangsheng practice, mindfulness is practised in everyday life. It is focused on cultivating healthy habits and abilities, such as learning the 'territory of the mind', in Dinah's terms, or learning to 'be where she is', for Lynn. It is entirely mundane, an ongoing daily practice of bringing intentional awareness to everyday activities in a particular way that for practitioners is explicitly associated with the cultivation of mental health and with living well much more broadly.

Thus, everyday life takes on non-ordinary meaning for mindfulness practitioners. Sheringham highlights (2006) that the everyday is transformed when too much value is attributed to it, either positively or negatively. Exploring interconnecting twentieth-century discourses about the everyday, Sheringham writes (ibid., 22) that

> any appeal to everydayness as interesting or valuable is likely to involve rehabilitation or exhortation: look at what you've overlooked! See the significance of the seemingly insignificant! Yet, in the sphere of the everyday, such zeal is paradoxical. If we go too far, the everyday ceases to be itself: it becomes the exceptional, the exotic, the marvellous. Transfigured, the commonplace is no longer commonplace.

For mindfulness practitioners, the everyday is both positively and negatively valued. Mindfulness practitioners highlight the negative consequences of living on 'autopilot'. The everyday develops as an intellectual and practical preoccupation both as a symptom of modern life and also as a rebellion against the functionalism or instrumentalism that it is thought to engender. This relies on a negative evaluation of non-reflective everyday life: that which leads to checking out, avoiding emotion or being disconnected from bodily sensations, as though 'ordinary' experience of the world is disconnected or misaligned. At the same time, everyday experience is positively valued as the locus of sacrality. It is the site at which one might return to 'wakefulness' by cultivating awareness in everyday activity. The veil of mundane experience may be lifted to reveal what Virginia Woolf described as 'moments of being' that originate *within* the sphere of the everyday. This positive valorisation of the everyday identifies it as the site for a return to value and meaning by engaging with it in a different way, in contrast to the impoverished 'everyday' of modern instrumentalism.

Negative views of everyday life as a blinkered habituation that numbs emotional awareness and positive valorisations of the everyday as the locus of sacrality both single the everyday out from the flow of life, and thus in both cases it no longer 'goes without saying'. Both the problem of 'automatic pilot', of 'sleepwalking' through the world without noticing it, and the transformative potential of learning to bring awareness to mundane activities are to be found in everyday life. In the attention to the everyday through awareness training, the practitioner 'tunes in' to that which is usually hidden by habit. Mindfulness comes close to Sheringham's characterisation of 'projects' which take the everyday as their object. In his examples, exercises such as intentionally noticing the frequency of specific unremarkable occurrences, or repeatedly describing the same scene on a particular section of a train journey, make projects of everyday activities. As he writes (2006, 391),

> By diverting attention from a goal to the carrying out of a repeated, preordained programme, the project creates its own intermediate spatiotemporal zone. In so doing, it generates attention to the present, to the unresolved matter of what is still in process (the process may be the spectator's current flow of awareness). The project is a frame, but nothing that comes to fill that frame can be said to complete or realize the project, which always remains open and unfinished. Yet within its framework a shift, essentially a shift of attention, takes place. The project brings us into proximity with something that might have seemed familiar, but which we now acknowledge more fully. In this sense we can see at work in the project the interface of alienation and appropriation that is central to thinking about the everyday.

Through the practice of awareness in otherwise habitual daily activities, practitioners seek to cultivate a reflective awareness of their own minds. Individual 'ordinary' activities (cleaning drawers, folding laundry) are singled out from the flow of everyday experience and become the site for the cultivation of awareness.

I have been arguing that mindfulness is world-affirming: through voluntary daily practice, ordinary experiences take on new meaning. This suggests that 'ordinary' and 'everyday' experience may sometimes be extraordinary, and may often be experienced as something other than 'everyday' because the ordinary and the everyday take on specific social significance and are embedded in broader ethical projects. Clarke (2014) has drawn a similar conclusion in his consideration of the 'ordinary ethics' of 'extraordinary' Sufi practices in Lebanon. He argues that miraculous practices of bodily mortification, 'aim to take one out of the ordinary. But the extraordinary does not therefore lie beyond the social; rather, it is constituted within it' (2014, 420).[2] In his ethnographic interrogation of ordinary and extraordinary experience, Clarke argues that extraordinary experience too has its ethics: its conventions, its responsibilities and virtues, its bodily and social techniques, its contradictions, its reasons and aesthetics. The more one scrutinizes the extraordinary, he claims, the more ordinary it becomes, and conversely, the more one examines everyday life, the less ordinary it appears: 'One does indeed end up by rendering "the strange familiar and the familiar strange", as the old saw runs' (ibid.). For mindfulness practitioners, engaging differently with ordinary experience offers both a means for finding meaning in life, a source of values, and also a means for living better within the 'maelstrom' of modernity (Berman 2009, 345). It ameliorates and valorises daily life, re-enchanting it by imbuing mundane activity with an un-ordinary quality of engagement. Awareness training offers a way of re-enchanting mundane experience and perceiving the immediacy of life in all of its extraordinary ordinariness.

From the Sublimey to the Corblimey

Despite the critique of unreflective everyday life and the neo-Romantic vital-ism of daily experience, both of which informed their practice, practitioners rarely described mindfulness to me as revolutionary or epiphanic, but rather as a perpetual 'return' to the work of being with or being near emotions as they unfold in the midst of life. They repeatedly drew my attention to the value of reflection itself when they spoke about practice. John told me that he now thinks of his relationship with his mind as a contract:

> We are relating to our mind and there's this to and fro that's happening. And I think 'Hang on, I have a say in this', it's not just this (pointing to his head) that goes off on its own and tells me how it's going to be and how I'm going to feel. It's like, 'Hang on, there's a contract here between you and I, we are in it together.

Similarly, I was told by Dave, who left a high-profile job as a journalist after experiencing a significant and terrifying period of depression and anxiety, and now works as a mindfulness teacher, that he feels he's found a wholly different way of approaching his own experiences of anxiety. He came to mindfulness as a mental health intervention at a very dark period of his life, and he describes his first experiences of mindful reflection as com-pletely new

> You can be present to what's happening in a way that's different to being caught unconsciously in it. And your thoughts don't have to define you. That was completely new for *me*, anyway.

This echoes what Taylor, in his magisterial account of modern identity (1989), refers to as 'radical reflexivity' to account for an increasing trend of 'standing back' from experience in order to remake oneself through disciplined work. 'What this calls for', he writes, 'is the ability to take an instrumental stance to one's given properties, desires, inclinations, tendencies, habits of thought and feeling, so that they can be *worked on'* (1989, 159–60; see also McMahan 2008, 201–2). Taylor continues (1989, 163),

Instead of being swept along to error by the ordinary bent of our experience, we stand back from it, withdraw from it, reconstrue it objectively, and then learn to draw defensible conclusions from it. To wrest control from 'our appetites and our preceptors,' we have to practice a kind of radical reflexivity. We fix experience in order to deprive it of its power, a source of bewitchment and error.

John's comments, that he has a relationship with his own mind, and that this 'contract' means that his mind doesn't 'tell him' how he's going to feel, are echoed in Dinah's comments, cited previously, that the danger of not having a relationship with her mind is that she will 'feel shit' and 'act out' when she is struggling. As we saw in the last chapter, mindfulness practitioners learn metacognitive theories and strategies (what people think about thinking, and what they think they should do about it), and these inform their efforts to cultivate habits and skills that will transform the ways in which life is experienced and understood. Practitioners are learning to theorise about and relate to their minds in particular ways, as they reflect on and attempt to act on their own minds and experiences. John's and Dinah's observations reflect a broader commitment to the idea that developing a metacognitive relationship with one's mind supports mental health and living well.

Practitioners understand the cultivation of present-focused metacognitive awareness both as a technique to support mental health at specific times and as an ongoing practice that informs life much more broadly. I was struck by this in my relationship with Marion. Marion had stumbled onto Buddhism at the age of nineteen, when she was working as a volunteer in Sri Lanka and did a ten-day meditation course which left a strong impression on her. Intermittently through her twenties she attended various meditation days, but when she was thirty-four she went on a retreat and began to re-engage seriously with the practice. Over the course of fifteen years she found meditation to be of enormous value to her, but was always aware that it was difficult to communicate to others why that was, and she felt a gap in conversations when she tried to explain to those who did not mediate why going on retreat could matter so much to her. 'Here's what I think,' said Marion, sitting in her sunlit garden. She paused, pursing her lips. I could hear a lawnmower from somewhere further down the terrace. 'What is a good life, anyway?' she asked. I had asked her why she practises mindfulness, and I was surprised by the sudden silence in our conversation. After what felt like a long time she said, 'So, if the practice has been a way to confront life with courage and honesty . . . and if mindfulness has been the best way I've found of doing that . . . just to make sure I'm saying this right. . . .' She paused again, looking up to the sky. 'So, the most meaningful way to live a life is with courage and honesty in that ongoing process of human development, and it's the development of wisdom and compassion.' Marion was now focused and looking me straight in the eye over the garden table. She reflected on what she had just said, telling me that she chose her words carefully because she did not want to use the word 'transformation'; she thought 'transformation' smacked of hubris. In her opinion, very few people ever really transform, and

> for the rest of us it seems to me it's a bit of a pottering path in which you hope you're heading in the right direction towards, you know, not repeating destructive patterns, towards trying to . . . anyway . . . that I think would be the meaning of the practice. And I think there is a very profound challenge in all of that.

Marion's description of her engagement with mindfulness as 'pottering' provides a fitting shorthand for its place in daily life for many practitioners. Mindfulness is both understood as profoundly important—a means to live with courage and honesty—and also an everyday component of a wider ethical life. 'To potter' suggests ambling, busying oneself in an agreeable way, or paying attention to small tasks at hand in an unhurried manner. People 'potter' around their garden sheds, for example. This ongoing attentional work is gentle and is found in daily life: washing the dishes, doing the laundry, drinking tea; and yet people consistently described it as 'profound'. Practitioners engage in intentional practices of self-reflection in everyday life and this impacts their relationships with others and with their own mental health. Marion and others consciously engage in practices such as mindfulness, through which they intentionally cultivate a particular form of self-awareness, an awareness that they hope will inform the ways in which they face the challenges of daily life. Marion's response reflects the—albeit differently articulated—views of Leslie and Lynn that mindfulness is both ordinary and profound. For similar reasons, Dinah marks her daily practice as important:

> This feels to me like the challenge of the human condition. What I stumble over again and again. If I think about my own anxiety, it still normally takes me a solid period of time with ruminative thoughts, before I go, 'Ah, here I am again, maybe I could do some practice.'

Dinah described an attitude of allowing as an important part of the relationship she had developed with herself. As she told me,

> I'm forty-nine next birthday and I don't feel grown up at all. And I think for me all those things that I've related to, the classic not being good enough, or feeling shame in me or regret, I think mindfulness has helped me really befriend them. And I'm so tender to those aspects of myself now, actually, rather than putting all the energy into keeping them locked away and unseen. Or catching a glimpse and not wanting them to be there, but instead, allowing them to be part of me. So, there is a huge allowing.

In their accounts of themselves, practitioners consistently emphasised the value of 'being with' difficult emotional experiences. For example, Lynn, who was single and in her late forties, worried that she had trouble meeting men:

> I guess I feel these things, like 'I'm going to be alone for the rest of my life, there must be something wrong with me' and I know it's not true, it's just a thought or a fear, but I am feeling it. And so, I don't want to really get into it and fuel it, but I don't want to pretend it's not there either, because it is, and I *am* feeling it. So, there's a balancing act of recognising it and allowing it to be there without either pushing it away or getting really into it.

Lynn's commitment to reflective awareness and an attitude of allowing as an ongoing practice was significant for her relationship with her thoughts. Similarly, Leslie described mindfulness as a way of relating differently to her 'stuff':

> When things come up, it's my old stuff, to do with abuse or being thrown into things at an early age, and when that stuff comes up that's great, I'm familiar with that territory, but then what do I do with that? Does the compassion to stuff that we're learning, the allowing, the kindness, does that let us go away with it and hold it? For me, yes. I know my patterns and I am very resilient.

Learning a metacognitive relationship that was 'allowing' was described as profound by practitioners, and yet it remained committedly located in ongoing everyday life.

Metacognition in the Extraordinary Ordinary

The ordinary and the everyday thus emerge as vital concepts in the ways in which people approach social life. For practitioners, they are informed by anxiety about the nature of unreflective life, a quasi-utopian valorisation of the everyday and a committed practice of treating habitual practices as a focus of attention. Mindfulness practitioners are concerned with what they identify as the everyday work of living well, in which the ordinary and the everyday take on specific meanings. Typically, these people are getting by in the mundane circumstances of family and work dynamics. The challenges of sick children, marital breakdown and mental health are understood by them to be the ordinary stuff of life. Engagement with mindfulness is similarly understood to be a daily practice of tending to one's own mind. This ongoing self-reflection is located in routine activities. It is highly quotidian, aimed not at transcendence, but at the experience of being with or being near 'ordinary' experience through metacognitive awareness; and yet, time and again, people described their mindfulness practice to me as 'profound'. Returning to mindfulness in the midst of life, we are presented with an intentional commitment to reflection: using everyday activities as the site for intentional awareness training, Marion actively seeks to relate to her own life in a particular way (with courage and honesty); Dinah befriends parts of herself that she feels uncomfortable with; and John upholds a contract with his mind. The practice of reflective awareness informs everyday life, occurring in the ways in which people experience the particularities of quotidian situated action. Bound up with the work of mindfulness is a broader valorisation of a healthy relationship with oneself as an important component of living well, achieved through an ameliorative world-affirming practice, that seeks to make 'extraordinary' experience of 'ordinary' occurrence.[3]

The mindfulness practitioners quoted in this chapter illustrate an argument on behalf of the everyday as both a dystopian aspect of modern life, but also as a bearer of significance. Understanding the everyday in relation to contemporary anxiety about mental health enables us to make sense of the positive and negative problematisation of the everyday more broadly. In the development of ordinary ethics, Lambek sought to find ways of accounting for shared human problems and concerns: 'how to live in the world; how to act; how to live and act *with (and as) others*; how to make and maintain commitments and how to balance or diverge from them; how to know with certainty; how to partition skepticism; how to go forward with care, hope, and enthusiasm; how to get through sorrow and experience joy' (Lambek 2016, 782; emphasis in original). Mindfulness practitioners reflect Lambek's questioning as they explicitly explore how to live well in the circumstances in which they find themselves. Mindfulness does not require special circumstances or parameters, and it is brought to bear on the most mundane of activities. In this context, it is committedly a 'how to' practice for engaging with ordinary life embedded in everyday practices as practitioners cultivate sensibilities within daily life, informed by a broader idea that living well entails cultivating a healthy relationship with one's own mind. Posed as a question, the need for such attention to mental health in the midst of life is driven by an anxiety that unreflective everyday modern life is misaligned or unhealthy. Far from being that which passes without comment, the everyday comes into focus as anxiety increases about mental ill-health. 'Everydayness' emerges from indeterminacy and is transformed in the process simultaneously transforming uneventful daily experience into the site of a problematic disengagement from life and offering the possibility of a re-engagement with the 'present moment'. It is thus possible not only that 'ordinary' and 'everyday' are not necessarily synonyms (see Clarke 2014; Kelly 2008; Sayeau 2013, 8), but that they are not ordinary or everyday, either.

The extraordinary uptake of mindfulness by people who have never suffered from depression cannot be accounted for only in terms of the prevention of mental ill-health. For many people mindfulness practice is a way of cultivating positive mental health as a constituent component of living well. Both positive and negative valorisation of the everyday may be understood as structural features of modernity, and as two sides of the same coin. As a response to the effects of modern life, the critique is itself profoundly shaped by modernity. It is not an outright critique of modernity as a whole, but rather of those features of modernity (such as emotional alienation) that are negatively valued. The positive Romantic values of the development of a subjective richness in its full affective depth and complexity (Löwy and Sayre 2001, 25) are informed by a melancholic nostalgia for a return 'home' and experience of loss in contemporary society. The Romantic valorisation of 'ordinary' life as the site of 'extraordinary' experience and wonder emerges in response to the 'tedious uniformization of life' (ibid., 35). Foucault argues (1997, 310) that modernity is often characterised as a discontinuity of time or a break with tradition, and that being modern

> lies in adopting a certain attitude with respect to this movement; and this deliberate, difficult attitude consists in recapturing something eternal that is not beyond the present instant, nor behind it, but within it [. . .]; modernity is the attitude that makes it possible to grasp the 'heroic' aspect of the present moment. Modernity is not a phenomenon of sensitivity to the fleeting present; it is the will to 'heroize' the present.

The present takes on a high value which is 'indissociable from a desperate eagerness to imagine it, to imagine it otherwise than it is, and to transform it not by destroying it but by grasping what it is'. This deliberate attitude of modernity is tied to an asceticism: 'To be modern is not to accept oneself as one is in the flux of passing moments; it is to take oneself as object of a complex and difficult elaboration' (ibid., 311). To be modern, for Foucault, is to engage in voluntary modes of relating to reality and ways of acting and behaving in a practice of liberty. Thus the modern subject is characterised by a critical ethos in which 'the critique of what we are is at one and the same time the historical analysis of the limits imposed on us and an experiment with the possibility of going beyond them' (ibid., 319). On these terms, mindfulness is supremely modern: informed by a critique of aspects of modernity while also offering a re-engagement with modern life by which practitioners might not just survive but thrive, mindfulness practice matters to people like John and Dinah because through it they develop a relationship with their own minds. The aim is not radically to transform the structures of modern political and social life, or to return to a prelapsarian, 'primitive' or 'traditional' past, but rather to live well within them. Practitioners voluntarily engage in practices of self-care through which they seek to ameliorate their experience of the world in which they find themselves. As Dave told me, 'The solution isn't getting out of this; it's trying to find a different way of being *with* it.' Practitioners think that the deleterious effects of modernity are experienced in the mind, and it is here, by developing the capacity to relate to the mind differently through awareness training, that these effects may be addressed. Mindfulness is ameliorative, brought into the rhythm of everyday life rather than a revolutionary (or reactionary) rejection of modernity itself.

Mental health emerges as a constituent aspect of modern life, woven into understandings of the everyday circumstances in which people find themselves. The quotidian takes on an interesting and non-ordinary value in the construction and emergence of a wider set of discourses on mental healthcare as a focus in daily life. The increasing emphasis on the encouragement of health, rather than just the prevention of illness, means that concern for mental health increasingly seeps into areas that are historically outside the purview of medicine, explicitly located in activities that are identified as ordinary and everyday. The way in which mindfulness practitioners understand mental health is informed by the relationship between everyday life, living well and the mind. The everyday is linked to an experience of modernity that privileges the unconscious and contributes to mental ill-health, and it is the site of aspirations to forms of wakefulness and attention associated with 'living well'.

4

Mindful Parliamentarians: Common Sense and Living Well

'WE'RE NOT TALKING one-in-four here. It's not just about people who are sick. It's about you and me. It's about being stressed about stress, daisy-chaining thoughts together at three in the morning. Why are we so mean to ourselves? What is wrong? We're the smartest of all the animal kingdom, no question. But we don't know how to manage our minds.' It is a Tuesday afternoon in January 2017, and I am in the Jubilee Room in the Houses of Parliament, Westminster, where comedian Ruby Wax is describing mindfulness and why it is needed to a smiling audience comprised of government ministers, parliamentarians from both the House of Commons and the House of Lords, special advisors and staff. Before leading the group in a practice, she says, 'Let me tell you what mindfulness is not, okay? It isn't saying hello to your dishes before you wash them, or standing naked in the rain smiling inanely, or getting insurance so you don't come back as a cockroach.' The assembled parliamentarians and Westminster staff obediently close their eyes and adjust their postures as Ruby guides them to focus their awareness on the sensations of breathing.

The purpose of the meeting is to encourage more parliamentarians to join one of the mindfulness courses offered in Westminster. One hundred and fifty parliamentarians have already completed a modified mindfulness course, and today's meeting is to be followed by the start of a new eight-week course, and a drop-in class for people who have already completed the course. Mark Williams and Ruby Wax are presenting today's meeting, and they make an unlikely double act. Williams is a softly spoken retired Oxford professor. He is one of the originators of MBCT (see chapter 2 above) and the former director of the Oxford Mindfulness Centre. In 2011 he adapted the framework of the MBCT course to make it available to non-clinical groups in his bestselling book already cited, *Mindfulness: A Practical Guide to Finding Peace in a Frantic World* (Williams and Penman 2011; hereafter *Frantic World*), upon which the courses in Westminster are based. The possibility offered by this volume is emancipatory: it provides an account of the human mind and modes of thinking, and a practical 'how to' for psychological self-practice, explaining to readers how they might learn to reduce negative, unhealthy or automatic thinking patterns. By 2017 it had maintained its place for six years in the Amazon Top Five list; to date, it has sold over 1.5 million copies and has been translated into twenty-five languages. It is designed as a self-directed course, with guided audio mindfulness practices narrated by the author. (Mindfulness teachers joke that Mark's soft Durham tones send more people to sleep around the world than counting sheep.)

Ruby Wax, by contrast, is a fast-talking midwest Jewish American. She is feisty, fiercely clever and very funny. As well as being a well-known actress and comedian, she holds a degree in psychology from Berkeley and a master's degree in MBCT from Oxford. She is a staunch campaigner on mental health and a leading advocate for mindfulness training. She speaks powerfully about her own mental health experiences, and she received an OBE in 2015 for her mental health campaigning. On this day, she is in a good mood. Her second book on mindfulness, *A Mindfulness Guide for the Frazzled*, has just come out and has maintained its position at number one for the second week running. The night before, she opened her stage tour, *Frazzled*. Part stand-up, part psychology lecture, part mindfulness practice, the show was to go on to sell out theatres around the country before returning to London for a month-long residency at the Leicester Square Theatre.

On the morning of this meeting, Ruby and I began in the café just inside the Cromwell Green entrance to the Houses of Parliament, sitting underneath television screens showing the then prime minister, Theresa May, standing on the steps of 10 Downing Street to announce her Brexit plan. Given the chronic political turmoil that characterised Britain at the time, the message that parliamentarians could reduce their levels of stress and anxiety by learning simple meditation techniques seemed like spitting into the wind. But large numbers of parliamentarians had completed the parliamentary mindfulness course, and there was significant appetite for more.

Working with parliamentarians who practise mindfulness, what emerged was an ethnographically specific valorisation of 'common sense' informed by popular psychology and private concerns about mental health and well-being.

In what follows, I first provide an account of the development of mindfulness courses for parliamentarians, and then examine the influence of popular psychology books—such as *Frantic World*—in the UK. Popular psychology books often convey an emancipatory message. They provide universalising accounts of the evolved nature of the mind and the ways in which humans think, choose and react. And, as in *Frantic World*, psychology forms the basis from which new strategies are advanced for countering the tendencies of automatic cognitive processes. I show that universalist ideas from the psychological sciences inform the ways in which people think about mental health and also the strategies that people employ to address it. I argue that the universalist message of popular psychology books is invested with specific ethical and political meaning as it is interpreted in different ways by different people. In the previous chapter, we saw that mindfulness therapists incorporate mindfulness practices into their daily lives, that they approach 'ordinary' experiences with mindful awareness and that they describe doing so as both pragmatic and profound. In this chapter, I focus on parliamentarians who have practised mindfulness as a support for mental health and as a way of living more fully. Parliamentarians described their mindfulness practice differently depending on whether they were applying it to their personal or their professional lives. When describing their personal experience of mindfulness, they spoke of the complications of navigating mental health, living well and ethical conduct. But when they spoke about mindfulness in their professional lives, they framed it as a pragmatic support for the stressful world of politics; practising mindfulness was just 'common sense'.

Popular psychology has influenced the uptake of mindfulness in popular culture, describing the ways in which cognition has evolved, the pan-human ability to take the self as an object of reflection, and the techniques by which people might learn to do so. But, I suggest, it is necessarily the case that the universalising principles of psychology are incorporated into the ways in which people understand themselves in culturally specific ways. In highlighting the social life of psychology, we are able to point to the accretion of cultural assumptions that shape the taken-for-granted nature of ongoing transformations in the category of mental health. Psychological knowledge has become a way of understanding human nature and ordering human experience on the basis of that understanding. But as people engage with knowledge from the psychological sciences, they invest it with their own values as they incorporate it into life in culturally specific ways.

Mindful Parliamentarians

The first mindfulness classes in the UK parliament began four years earlier as an initiative developed by Chris Ruane, the then Labour MP for the Vale of Clwyd in north Wales, and Richard Layard, a senior economist at the London School of Economics and Political Science (LSE) and Labour peer (member of the House of Lords). Chris had come across mindfulness while seeking to address the effects of long-term unemployment in his constituency. This predominantly rural area had been hit by grinding unemployment for a variety of reasons, including the decline of tourism, government austerity measures and the collapse of local industry. Chris had been active in implementing a range of social and economic interventions to support the regeneration of the area, and he promoted mindfulness for job seekers as they weathered the effects of long-term unemployment. He told me that chronic unemployment impacts income and consumption patterns, family relations and re-employability, but that it also has profound effects on physical and mental health. And he thought that depression and anxiety are strong predictors of future job and income losses, contributing to a vicious cycle of unemployment and under-employment: people who are unemployed for longer than a year are likely to face mental health challenges which compound the structural challenges of finding employment. For this reason, Chris thought, it was important that his constituents receive psychological support, and he began to investigate whether mindfulness would be appropriate. He organised the first debate about mindfulness in parliament in December 2012, focusing on unemployment. He described his motivation to me as simple: he needed to find cost-effective ways to help his constituents get back into work.

A confidential mental health report had recently been commissioned in Westminster, which detailed the rates of depression and anxiety amongst politicians.[1] On the back of the mindfulness and unemployment debate, Chris wondered if introducing short mindfulness courses for politicians might provide a helpful redress to the high levels of anxiety self-reported in the Westminster report. He bumped into Richard Layard in a corridor and began a conversation about mindfulness classes for politicians. Lord Layard had produced the influential 'Depression Report' in 2006 (LSE 2006), which led to the establishment of the Improving Access to Psychological Therapies (IAPT) programme by the Department of Health (see Pollock 2009). IAPT is an NHS programme of services across England that offers interventions and clinical training in therapeutic techniques approved by the National Institute of

Health and Care Excellence (NICE) for treating people with depression and anxiety disorders.[2] Sometimes referred to as the UK government's 'Happiness Tsar' (Jeffries 2008) because of his work in 'happiness economics', Layard has promoted mindfulness-based therapies as one possible corrective to the high levels of self-reported unhappiness and worrying epidemiological statistics on the rise in mental health diagnoses (see chapter 6 below), and he had previously commended mindfulness-based interventions as 'mind training' (Layard 2005, 189). Chris Ruane and Richard Layard contacted Mark Williams, who was then the head of the Oxford Mindfulness Centre, and Chris Cullen, a senior mindfulness teacher and the co-founder of the Mindfulness in Schools Project, in December 2012 to discuss the possibility of holding mindfulness courses for parliamentarians.

The first mindfulness course in parliament began on the 17 January 2013. The course was promoted as a skills training programme, rather than a form of therapy, and the course leader was referred to as a 'teacher' rather than a 'therapist'. It was felt that this distinction would make it more appealing for people to attend. Early courses were held under the promise of strict anonymity, but once the media learned about the initiative, it began to receive coverage. This marked the beginning of the British media cycle around mindfulness to which I turn in the Conclusion of this book. Journalists wanted to know what the courses were and how they were funded—was the taxpayer subsidising therapy for MPs? The response to each enquiry was clear: the courses were a form of skills training rather than a therapeutic intervention; they were being offered by a charity, the Oxford Mindfulness Foundation, which supports the Oxford Mindfulness Centre, and while politicians were encouraged to make a donation towards them, this was not mandatory. By the launch of the All-Party Parliamentary Group (APPG) in May 2014 (see chapter 5), eighty-five parliamentarians had completed the course. Chris Ruane noted that an initial hesitancy about 'creating a cult in parliament' had shifted, and increasing numbers of people from all parties were enrolling on the courses, though they were still the subject of some gentle mockery: 'I have friends who come by and say "Om",' he remarked.

Classes were based on the course laid out in *Frantic World* and were kept brief: a 'short-course drive-through version of mindfulness', as one teacher described it. As of July 2022, the courses are still running. They are taught in groups of eight to twelve people, led by a trained mindfulness teacher, that meet once a week for seventy-five-minute sessions over an eight-week period. As with the MBCT course for clinical populations that was the focus of chapter 2 above, the *Frantic World* course is built up from a series of intentional exercises, including mindfulness of breath, mindful movement, a body scan and mindful eating, as well as intentionally bringing an attitude of kindly awareness to everyday activities such as doing the washing up, eating or bathing. Each session is followed by 'homework'—guided mindfulness practices that participants listen to at home, and bringing mindful awareness to specified routine activities. Some practices from the MBCT course, such as keeping pleasant- and unpleasant-event calendars, or completing a depressive relapse signature chart or an action plan, are not included in the *Frantic World* course. The *Frantic World* course also includes practices that are not present in the MBCT course, such as a homework task in week six to perform a random act of kindness each day.

The Virtue Ethics of Cognitive Psychology

The *Frantic World* book provides an overview of the cognitive framework for depression and anxiety, and a truncated version of the eight-week clinical MBCT programme for readers. It is designed as a practical guide to mindfulness for people who are experiencing stress and anxiety, but who have not received a clinical diagnosis. In *Frantic World*, experiences of depression and anxiety are explained as effects of the relationship between pan-human evolved cognitive capacities and the nature of the world in which we live. As we saw in chapter 2 above, the cognitive model of emotional regulation and depressive relapse is premised on an understanding that human cognitive functioning has evolved a highly developed problem-solving capacity that, while very useful in task-oriented movement through the world, is maladaptive when applied to emotional problems for which no immediate solution is present. The day-to-day experiences of stress, anxiety and depression, shorthanded by Ruby Wax's descriptor 'frazzled', can be ameliorated through a course of mindfulness, and the practices in the book are to be incorporated into daily life in order to 'tackle anxiety and to rediscover a love of life' (Williams and Penman 2011, 2).

The runaway success of *Frantic World*, and its influence in making mindfulness a household term, cannot be underestimated, and it reflects the crossover popularity of publications from the psychological sciences more broadly. Popular interest in psychological work has centred on theories which propose that much of our thinking occurs automatically, is conditioned by bias, or is 'primed' by situational factors. These vary from smells, ambient noise and the circumstances that immediately precede moral choice (see Merrit, Doris and Harman 2010). For example, American social psychologist Jonathan Haidt's bestselling work, in books such as *The Happiness Hypothesis* (2006) and *The Coddling of the American Mind* (Lukianoff and Haidt 2018), exposes 'traditional wisdom to the scrutiny of modern science', arguing that moral judgements are often made automatically, and that moral reasoning is post-hoc (see also Haidt 2001). Relatedly, Daniel Kahneman's massively influential book *Thinking, Fast and Slow* (2011) advanced a dual-purpose paradigm of thinking. 'System 1' is easily triggered, based on brief impressions, intuitions and feelings. 'System 2' is reflective, more deliberative and requires concentration. 'Fast' modes of thinking are influenced by hindsight bias, the inability to recognise 'sunk costs', the tendency to misremember, based on how things ended, and a tendency to discount risk. Similarly, Richard Thaler and Cass Sunstein's highly influential bestseller *Nudge* (2008) draws on insights from the behavioural sciences to argue that the human mind is fallible. Humans are 'loss averse', and often discount thoughts of the future when making decisions. Furthermore, decisions are 'anchored' on salient pieces of information, and as such can be 'primed' by new or recently received information, or by the immediate environment.[3] In each of these examples, people who might think of themselves as having the capacity to make judgements about the right thing to do are revealed to be acting (to varying degrees) as a result of psychological mechanisms and situational cues (see also Doris 2002; Alfano 2013). Moral autonomy and deliberation are revealed to be fronts for hardwired or automatic processes, of which people are often unaware.

In each of these cases, experience and choice result from human psychology rather than moral education or moral character; we are revealed to be not the deliberative moral agents that we take ourselves to be. Decision-making is no longer the preserve of character in any sense of Aristotelian virtue ethics. At first blush the conclusion from this appears to amount to a form of moral deflation—our responses, emotions or thoughts are not the result of cultivated moral character, but are rather the reactions of automatic hardwired processes that are increasingly triggered by the structures of modernity. But as Anderson (2018) has highlighted, the crossover popularity of modern psychology is in many ways crypto-moral. The principle that underpins each of these theories, and part of the explanation for their uptake in popular and policy circles, is emancipatory: a normative investment in the idea that the better we understand these pan-human dispositions, the better able we might be to correct for them. Kahneman believes (2011) that educating organisations and institutions about the dangers of problematic thinking can provide a regulatory oversight to practices. Similarly, Thaler and Sunstein hold (2008) that understanding the psychological parameters of decision-making contexts and ingrained human biases can make it easier to 'nudge' people into choosing what is best for them. And Haidt proposes (2001, 829) that, given his findings, one can 'try to create a culture that fosters a more balanced, reflective, and fair-minded style of judgment'.

Once the ways in which our minds work have been delineated, it becomes sensible to ameliorate the more negative and automatic processes that inform our day-to-day emotional experiences, decision-making and assumptions. Popular psychology books, such as those just cited, promote a commitment to the idea that humans have the capacity to modify patterns of behaviour that are thought of as in some sense innate. Patterns of thinking and decision-making are thought to be to some extent hardwired and automatic, but it is also claimed that humans have the capacity to change the behaviour that feeds these patterns, and therefore need not be controlled by pan-human cognitive mechanisms. We are less ourselves than we think we are, but we can engage in practices which counter or make up for the effects of automatic processes or unwitting biases. Anderson argues that, in this way, popular psychology 'makes appeal to a conception of transformative self-awareness that is part of the long tradition of the examined life at the heart of virtue ethics and, more narrowly, Kantian [ethics] as well' (2018, 30). The findings of psychological and behavioural sciences are used as the basis from which to advocate for the formation of positive habits, 'a kind of retraining, or a willed affiliation with social contexts that will be formative of desirable moral habits ingrained over time' (ibid., 27). In this understanding, pan-human cognitive capacities become the site at which the work of character or virtue takes place. In this perspective, the idea that forms of virtue are learned depends on a particular universalising idea of human cognition (see Sherman 1989, 7). In each of the examples above, the insights of the psychological sciences account for human behaviour, reactions and choice, and human psychology is characterised as driven by flaws in human cognition. By providing practices and environments through which people can learn about and relate differently to their own minds, they might address and correct for these tendencies. Thus, universalist ideas about human psychology inform how people think about mental health and what they ought to do about it.

As we have seen, the authority and popularity of psychology in Britain have significantly influenced the ways in which mindfulness has been taken up in popular culture. The findings of the psychological sciences are articulated through popular psychology books that explain both why we feel the ways that we feel or make the choices that we do and, importantly, what we can do about it. The 'you' that is the focus of mindfulness practice, and is amenable to self-directed intervention, is not the story you tell about yourself or your messy history, it is not your synapses or genetic dispositions, and it is certainly not your depression. Rather, what is learned through self-help and non-clinical training in mindfulness is understood as a pan-human ability to take the self as an object of reflection while cultivating attitudinal dispositions of non-judgement and compassion. As we saw in Ruby Wax and Mark Williams's presentation in Westminster, mindfulness is premised on a cognitive and evolutionary model of mind. The unhelpful patterns of ruminative thought and problem solving which, while useful in the practicalities of life, are maladapted to the experience of emotion are destructive but powerful traps that contribute to stress, anxiety and depression. Cognitive functioning might be supported by learning to sit with and relate differently to experience without trying to fix or change it.

Common Sense and Living Well

Given the intensification of psychological subjectivity, and the parallels between 'the personal projects of individuals to live a good life' (Rose 1990, 10, 51) and political agendas (see chapter 5 below), part of the work of this chapter is to examine what people see as amenable to human intervention and what they understand as constraint—that is, what they can change or work on and what is given; deciding the answer to that is an ethical question. This reflects Kuan's theory of an 'ethics of trying' in her consideration of parenting in China. As she writes (2015, 18), an ethics of trying 'is a variety of moral experience that has less to do with conforming to normative moral codes than with a kind of practical philosophy, which takes causation and efficacy, responsibility and blame, as its central concerns'. Kuan draws out, in theoretical argument and ethnographic focus, the ways in which parents seek opportunities for action embedded in existing circumstances that they seek to work with, rather than against. As she writes of parenting in China (ibid., 61), 'parental intensity expresses a kind of moral agency that takes timely and situationally appropriate effort as a crucial element of being efficacious in this world'. An ethics of trying is reflected in the culturally specific ways in which parliamentarians describe how their mindfulness practice related to their professional lives. They were not seeking to change their professional world through their personal meditation practice (though as we shall see in chapter 5, this was clearly the focus of policy discussion about mindfulness); rather, they were seeking to live well within that world.

In her presentation about mindfulness in the Jubilee Room, Ruby begins by telling us that stress is evolutionarily advantageous: without it 'we'd all be in the Darwinian graveyard'; but that being 'frazzled' is different: being 'frazzled is being stressed about stress'. Stress kept us alive on the savannah: if a predator approaches a gazelle, a rush of cortisol and adrenaline provides the gazelle with the 'oomph' it needs to find safety. But, Ruby says, once it has escaped a lion attack, the gazelle goes back to grazing; 'it doesn't go on antidepressants'. In contrast, stress about stress—being 'frazzled'—is a new phenomenon, but one that results from our psychological make up. The problem, she tells us, is that we are besieged by bad news, and the effect on our bodies is the same whether the danger is behind us, or twenty thousand miles way; humans are creatures of addiction, and nothing is encouraging us to switch off. Ruby is followed by Mark, who emphasises that mindfulness has 'escaped the clinic' and entered popular culture. Everyone, from *Glamour Magazine* to mental health trusts, is talking about mindfulness. One consequence of this, as Mark sees it, is that mental health is being destigmatised: 'Someone can say, "I'm doing a mindfulness course," and no one bats an eyelid.' Mark believes that mindfulness might help large numbers of people manage their stress but, he says, it is not for everyone, and practising mindfulness 'shouldn't be a should'. For the room of assembled parliamentarians, Mark and Ruby present mindfulness as an ameliorative technique for the world of high stress, which enables a 'richer, fuller appreciation of life'.

A few things about this characterisation of mental health are worth drawing out. Mark and Ruby frame mental health as something of which every person can take care: learning to relate to the mind in a particular way, on purpose, is presented as beneficial for everybody, whether or not they have a history of mental health issues. This, it is argued, is because of the way in which the human mind is structured and how it responds to the world around it. In short, we must all take care of our minds, because of their very nature, and doing so will have positive effects on our experiences of the world. In the current injunction to cultivate a metacognitive relationship with one's own mind, a capacity for

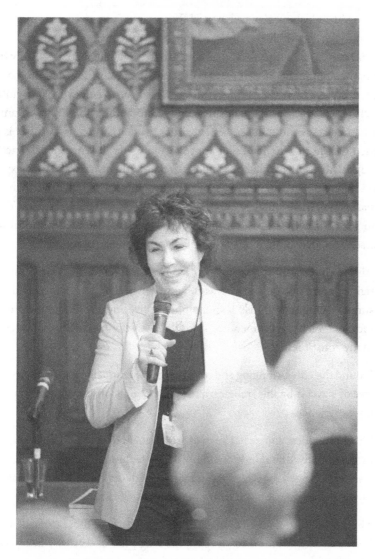

FIGURE 3. Ruby Wax teaching parliamentarians about mindfulness,
Westminster, January 2017. Photograph by Shai Dolev.

awareness is encouraged and valorised. Mark's comment that mindfulness has
'escaped the clinic' could not be truer. As is reflected in parliamentarians' participation in mindfulness courses, concern about mental health is no longer
limited to clinical populations, and relating to the mind in a particular way is
broadly understood to be 'good to do'. The stigma of mental illness (depression
and anxiety at least) is slipping away as it becomes increasingly normal for

people to think about themselves and their experiences in such terms. In response to this, mindfulness is imbued with both instrumental and ethical value. On the one hand, it is presented as ameliorative and pragmatic. As Ruby tells the parliamentarians, 'it isn't sitting on a gluten-free cushion'. Mindfulness is framed as a sensible redress to the stress that occurs when evolved cognitive structures rub up against the business end of modernity. It becomes common sense to practise mindfulness. On the other hand, mindfulness practice is intended to lead to a 'richer, fuller appreciation of life'. It is an ethical practice through which parliamentarians intend to relate to themselves and their experiences differently in order to 'rediscover a love of life'.

Parliamentarians publicly described mindfulness as a pragmatic and 'common sense' practice. For example, those who had attended mindfulness courses provided anonymous testimonials about their experience:

Although initially sceptical, [. . .] having completed the course, and attended every session, I'm a convert. It's just logical that we could all do with simple techniques to help us remember to live and appreciate the present moment. I'll be recommending it to all those who work with young people in my constituency.

I found the ethos, thinking and practice totally compelling and additionally, free of 'psycho-babble', religion and spiritual allusions. A very, very enriching experience.

The mindfulness course has been of great benefit to me both personally and professionally. The mindfulness breathing techniques and practical exercises have helped me to cope much better with the stresses and strains of a highly demanding job and gain a better work–life balance.

Mindfulness need not be thought of only as a 'cure' for those in need; it also helps one to know how to [. . .] enjoy living a life of service. I have found the mindfulness course amazingly helpful.

In today's mad world, a few well-earthed, indeed profoundly common sense, contemplative insights are truly invaluable.

In public discussion at Westminster, mindfulness was valued as a pragmatic tool for addressing garden-variety daily challenges, a down-to-earth measure for supporting practitioners as they navigate in-the-midst-of-life decisions and interactions (in the rather particular workplace of Westminster). As Geertz writes (1975, 7), 'common sense rests its [case] on the assertion that it is not a case at all, just life in a nutshell. The world is its authority.' But 'common sense' has a double meaning in this instance: it is simultaneously used to point to that which any sensible person would conclude, presented with sufficient information, and it signals good and practical judgement. 'Common sense' itself is valorised in the practical meaning that mindfulness holds for parliamentarians.

Yet, if in their professional lives parliamentarians valued mindfulness as a pragmatic and commonsensical tool, in their personal lives their engagement with it reflected a far broader ethical and emotional commitment. For example, in an interview, a senior Labour MP told me about the perspective that he thought mindfulness brought to his life. Peter had attended the mindfulness sessions from the beginning. Sitting together under the bombproof atrium of Portcullis House, opposite the Palace of Westminster, in 2016, he reflected on what had drawn him to meditation. For Peter, meditation was not primarily a way of dealing with anxiety or stress, although he thought that this was important. For him, meditation was a 'boon':

> It's the question that mankind's asked since the first time that he or she looked into a fire. It's in every wisdom tradition. What is a good and meaningful life? How do we connect with others and the environment? First you must connect with yourself, and mindfulness helps you do that. It helps you make better personal and professional decisions, no matter what your profession.

This interaction between personal and professional experience was reflected further in the ways in which parliamentarians understood mental health. A few days before the launch of the APPG (6 May 2014; see chapter 5), Tracey Crouch, a Conservative MP who had been through the course, 'came clean' about her mental health experience in an interview on the BBC Radio Four magazine programme *Woman's Hour*. She told the audience that she had been prescribed antidepressants, but she had been reluctant to take them and that she had joined the parliamentary classes as an alternative way of coping with her mental health problems. The interviewer, Jane Garvey, asked her whether speaking about this on the radio was part of a broader cultural shift in how we think about mental health: 'In some ways though, we are making strides, aren't we? The fact that you as an MP are prepared to admit that you've been prescribed antidepressants, that you've been interested in and taken part in mindfulness, I'm not sure that this would have happened five or six years ago, even.' Tracey responded,

> I don't like to admit it, to be honest with you. It was a particularly low period in my life and I think the problem with being an MP is that you have very much a public persona and a private persona and if you saw me in public at the beginning of last year you wouldn't think that there was anything wrong with me; but sometimes you just need a little bit of assistance and certainly mindfulness has helped me focus.

A few days later, at the launch of the APPG, Tracey told the assembled group that she had been commended in the corridors for her 'very brave confession of mental health issues' on national radio, which she had translated as political-speak for 'Congratulations on your act of professional suicide.' But, she maintained, if she was prepared to speak about her mental health experience then maybe others would be too. For Tracey, speaking about her mental health and mindfulness practice was part of a broader process of destigmatisation, one that she worried Westminster was not ready for, but that she was committed to, nonetheless. Her motivation for practice was her own mental health, and she saw her public confession of this as an important contribution to destigmatisation more broadly, but she also thought of mindfulness as a practical support for her professional life. She told the APPG that mindfulness helps her in her day-to-day life as a politician, and that she takes her shoes off as a way to 'ground' herself during Prime Minister's Questions.[4]

After Ruby Wax and Mark Williams's presentation in 2017, three parliamentarians commented publicly that they felt that mindfulness classes in Westminster had fostered friendships across the political spectrum and made Westminster a much friendlier place to work. For example, Lord Alan Howarth of Newport, a former Labour MP and government minister, closed the day by commenting that he had benefited from mindfulness and that it had changed his interactions with others:

> I started to attend the mindfulness classes four years ago [. . .]. This political world of ours, this political life of ours can perhaps, we love it, but it is a little crazy, isn't it? It's kind of hectic. It's stressful and stress is a very good thing, but you can get frazzled. And I think for me this weekly 'drop in' class as we call it, this weekly group is just an oasis of trust and friendship, something very important in our adversarial politics. It's a place where people of all parties come together. For me personally it is a great help to recuperate

my focus, my energy, my perspective, my sense of proportion, and my balance; to find a bit of calm.

In interviews with members of the two Houses, this view was qualified somewhat, however, with members commenting that while they valued a sense of support within the mindfulness group, politics was combative, and it would be unreasonable to think that that would change. As a former Liberal Democrat minister told me as we took tea in the tea-room in the House of Lords a few weeks later, 'This place is set up for opposition. Mindfulness helps me be well within that.' Nonetheless, she said, mindfulness was far more than just a pragmatic tool. She attributed feeling happier and more settled in herself to her meditation practice; each day she noted her emotional experience on a chart that she kept next to her desk, and this daily practice of awareness supported her sense of well-being.

A Neuroscientist in Westminster

On its own terms, popular psychology claims to offer insights into pan-human psychological processes of deliberation, choice and emotion. Tracing the social life of psychological ideas, however, it is possible to consider the culturally specific ways in which universalising psychological principles are interpreted and incorporated into how people understand themselves. As psychological knowledge travels, it is interpreted in diverse ways by different people, and is reinscribed with specific ethical and political meaning. By examining the social life of psychology, we might account for the meaning that people attribute to practices, organisational structures and ideas, and we might uncover the internalisation of values, the development of social imaginaries and the aspirations that motivate engagement with practices. For example, Matza's thorough ethnography of post-Soviet Russia (2018) shows that the work of psychologists in St. Petersburg is anchored in a complex universe of social meaning and relationships. Popular psychological practices emerged in Russia at the same time as the dynamic political transformations of the post-Soviet period, as citizens and psychologists reimagined both the nature of 'self' and the terms of political and social life through new psychotherapeutic modalities. Similarly, Long demonstrates (2013) that achievement psychology in Kepri province, Indonesia, is highly politicised. Measures of achievement incorporate the cultivation of 'human development' or 'well-being' sometimes framed by a neoliberal rhetoric of encouraging individuals to 'fulfil their potential', sometimes framed in the utilitarian terms of a 'motivated workforce'. As the nation seeks to compete in the 'global knowledge economy' the psychology of achievement has powerful consequences for how 'achievers' understand themselves and engage with the world. Comparatively, Hoesterey considers (2016) the ways in which popular psychology is merged with understandings of marital intimacy, Muslim piety and economic aspiration in Indonesia through his examination of the rise and fall of Aa Gym, a prominent Indonesian self-help guru. Aa Gym and other Muslim television preachers draw on the global psychological sciences, but also offer an Islamic corrective to what they see as the latter's secular foundations. The combination of piety and prosperity in Aa Gym's teaching and the exemplar of his own carefully crafted public image appeals to the aspirations and anxieties of middle-class Indonesian Muslims. Here, the combination of Muslim piety with popular psychology is presented as providing 'practical "how-to" knowledge of applying Islamic teachings to everyday life' (Hoesterey 2016, 11). Diverse forms of psychological knowledge are transformed into everyday wisdom and aspirational piety as middle-class Indonesians seek to achieve success through ethical comportment and the moral psychology of the heart.

While psychology tells a universalising story about our minds and the nature of suffering, this is incorporated into how people think about themselves and how they think they ought to respond to life in socially and culturally specific ways, as it is imbued with values, aspirations and ethics. As McMahan and Braun argue of mindfulness (2017, 15), '[b]olstered at each turn by scientific legitimation, [mindfulness] practice becomes enfolded in the wider landscape of metaphysics, moral values, and ways of being in the world'. As psychology travels, it shapes the taken-for-granted nature of phenomena in the world in culturally specific ways.

Parliamentarians' commitments to common sense and living well were reflected in the qualified way in which they engaged with a visiting American neuroscientist, Dan Siegel, who came to Westminster to talk about mindfulness and 'interpersonal neurobiology' in February 2019. Based in California, Siegel is a clinical professor of psychiatry at the UCLA School of Medicine and the executive director the Mindsight Institute. His work focuses on interpersonal neurobiology, but he is best known for his collaborations with the Dalai Lama and his books for general readers. *Mind: A Journey to the Heart of Being Human* (2016) and *Brainstorm: The Power and Purpose of the Teenage Brain* (2014) were both *New York Times* bestsellers. His most recent book, *Aware: The Science and Practice of Presence* (2018), integrated interpersonal neurobiology and mindfulness. He was in Westminster to talk about the neuroscience of meditation, and the Jubilee Room was packed again, with the front two rows taken up by parliamentarians, and the rest of the audience made up of parliamentary staff and civil servants.

Siegel's work is part of a second area of popular literature on meditation, this time coming from the neurological sciences. A slew of popular books has been published on the neuroscience of meditation (for example, Arden 2010; Culadasa (Yates) and Immergut 2015; Goleman and Davidson 2018; Lucas 2013; Siegel 2007), which, like the popular psychology books discussed earlier, argue both that humans are hardwired in certain ways and that we can do something about it. The effects of mindfulness practice are rendered visible through brain imaging, and mindfulness seemingly visibly changes the shape of the brain. For example, Hölzel and colleagues' work (Hölzel, Carmody et al. 2011; Hölzel, Lazar et al. 2011) using brain imaging appeared to demonstrate that an eight-week MBSR mindfulness meditation programme made measurable changes to the brain in the areas associated with memory, sense of self, empathy and stress. This study is frequently cited as the first 'best evidence' to demonstrate that meditation leads to changes in the brain's grey matter. Britta Hölzel said of her work, 'It is fascinating to see the brain's plasticity and that, by practicing meditation, we can play an active role in changing the brain and can increase our well-being and quality of life' (McGreevey 2011). Mindfulness now is not only consonant with science; it *is* scientific, and it can be employed as a technique to achieve scientifically measurable ends, be they neurological, psychological or both.[5] For example, Hanson writes (2009, 13) that mindfulness 'involves the skilful use of attention to both your inner and outer worlds. Since your brain learns mainly from what you attend to, mindfulness is the doorway to taking in good experiences and making them part of you.'

The suggestion is clear: our brains are available for intervention and meditation is a technology for taking control of and responsibility for the changes that occur. Both the ability to map brain states and theories of neuroplasticity provide validation for sustained meditation practice, as the evidence from the neurological and psychological sciences is incorporated into broader understandings of virtue, self-cultivation and living well. As Rose and Abi-Rached write (2013, 16), 'we are urged to recognize not only that our brains shape us, but also that we can and should act on our brains through our conscious decisions: reshaping our brains to reshape ourselves'. Underpinning this is an 'often unacknowledged intertwining of promises, hopes, anticipations, expectations and speculations' and these 'play a key role in shaping contemporary regimes of truth about persons and their mental lives' (ibid., 20). In this reading, virtue, mindfulness and wisdom are the foundation of personal growth and emotional well-being, and these are reflected in the neural and psychological functions of regulation, learning and selection. The conclusion from this is that you can 'use your mind to change your brain and benefit your mind' (Hanson 2009, 18).

Standing behind a microphone at the front of the room at Westminster, Dan Siegel was a fluent and engaging speaker. He began by asking who in the room had a regular reflective, contemplative or meditative practice and almost everyone put their hands up. Dan told us that like all complex systems, humans self-regulate their own becoming and he delineated four facets of mind (subjective experience, consciousness, information processing and self-organisation). He was at pains to highlight that none of these is limited to the brain, and that the mind, relationships and the embodied brain interact through energy and information. Linking different parts of this complex system optimises the mind, a process Dan referred to as 'integration'. He told us that the best way to encourage integration is through the 'three pillars of mind training': focused attention, open awareness and kind intention can all be trained, and when they are developed the brain is more integrated. The brain, he informed us, has two states: a reactive state (characterised by fight, flight, freeze and faint) and a receptive state (characterised by social engagement with others and with our own internal worlds), and that experience changes the structure of the brain. As he said, 'where attention goes, neural firing flows, and neural connection grows'. Dan led the audience in a mindfulness practice to illustrate the sketch of the mind that he had laid out, and everyone willingly participated. 'It's like cleaning your teeth every day,' he told us. 'Just as you have dental hygiene from brushing your teeth, this is mental hygiene for essentially strengthening your mind.'

Dan then moved on to the potential of neurological training for parliamentarians, stating that integrative training can provide a way for them to deal with political disagreement. He told us that in government, in families and in organisations nothing is achieved if people go into reactive states: 'Mindfulness is the most integrated technique you can practice,' he said. 'It's about how you comport yourself when you talk about Brexit.' According to Dan, parliamentarians could cultivate the experience of being aware and, by so doing, drop into the open space of a 'plane of possibility', and he exhorted the assembled parliamentarians to train their governmental officials so that they could guide the rest of the world:

> When you learn to live from the plane of possibility, you start to live with the reality that life is more like a verb than a noun. If you do this as parliamentarians you move to a world of creativity and innovation, you stay receptive not reactive. Open awareness is maximal uncertainty, a synonym for possibility and freedom.

Dan told his audience that integration leads to the insight that we are all part of the same whole and that the separate self is a delusion perpetuated by modern culture. By practising mindfulness, parliamentarians could move 'from a separate me to an integrated "Mwe"'.

In his short talk, Dan summarised some fairly complicated neurobiology and psychology, laying out a theory of the relationship between meditation practice and the brain, and the consequences of this for engagement with the world and with politics. But in the question-and-answer session that followed, it was clear that his audience endorsed his argument in a qualified way: they liked the neuroscience and the practice, and were excited by the possibilities that both held out for their personal lives. Where they pulled back, however, was when it came to the implications of this for a broader relational field of transformation. For example, a member of the House of Lords commented,

> Sitting here, it's wonderful to hear you speak. I'm a strong supporter of mindfulness in parliament but in practical politics a premium is put on certainty. If I disagree with a politician and want to challenge him or her then I need to be certain of my position. What you've said makes a lot of sense in terms of my own practice, but I don't see how to turn that into being an effective politician.

Another question from a member of the House of Lords highlighted engagement with neuroscience and the challenges of political structure: 'It's an adversarial system, and the press love blood on the carpets. For example, how could this contribute to alternative arrangements for the Irish backstop?'[6] Dan responded that a more integrated approach to politics might enable unexpected possibilities: 'Creative solutions will come from these halls and blow the world away', he said, 'if politicians are integrated.' But, while his neurological insights into personal meditation practice were welcomed, Dan's call for a transformation of political culture met with some scepticism. This was reflected the next day in an email from the volunteers who had organised the event, which read,

> [Dan's] proposal that integration underpins the benefits of mindfulness practice, as well as the health of the brain, individuals and society, provides an inspiring meta-narrative for those of us working to develop any of them. Whether or not future research validates the theory connecting neuroscience with contemplative practice and quantum physics exactly as it was presented to us, I hope you agree that it was fascinating food for thought!

I take the 'whether or not' phrasing of this to be a politely British way to say that 'we're with you (only) up to a point'. The talk was very well attended and received, but the way in which it was responded to reflects the values of the audience: in their personal lives they found meaning in mindfulness practice but this did not mean that they were seeking to transform political life; instead mindfulness offered a pragmatic support for people working in a stressful and adversarial professional culture.

Conclusion: The Social Life of Psychology

An ethnographic focus on the popularity of psychological knowledge highlights heterogeneity in the ways in which people engage with it, how they understand themselves in relation to it and how they embed it in the moral projects through which they engage with the world. Writing of mindfulness in America, Wilson reports (2014, 110) that it 'moves from being taught in clinical situations to being discussed in books for general consumption, and soon enough techniques for the management of severe pain and crippling psychological issues are applied to the ordinary aches, frustrations, and stresses of contemporary life'. But whereas in America mindfulness 'is mainstreamed by being adapted to make the lives of [. . .] harried hockey dads and soccer moms better, one mindfully eaten cookie at a time' (ibid., 105), in Westminster engagement with meditation practice is simultaneously instrumental and ethical. It is framed as a tool for navigating stressful working environments without becoming 'frazzled' and also as a personal 'way of being', a boon and a cultivated reflective relationship with parliamentarians' emotional lives. People engage with psychological knowledge as they seek to ameliorate their lives in pragmatic and ethical ways in the midst of the circumstances in which they find themselves, whether that be family relationships, the corridors of Westminster or, as we shall see in the next chapter, in hospitals, prisons and schools.

The interpretation of mental health represented here reflects a broader trend towards a destigmatisation and a universalist reframing of mental health in the UK. As a preventative intervention, mindfulness is understood to be universally applicable. It is based on a universalist theory of mind and mental suffering, whereby it is presented as relevant for all people, whether or not they have ever received a mental health diagnosis. In this chapter, I hope to have highlighted the shift in scale between the universal and the particular. Here, the 'meta-narrative' of the psychological sciences makes this shift look natural: it becomes commonsensical to take care of one's mental health. This rests on an ethnographically specific valorisation of common sense and a clear effort to work within, rather than transform, the structures in which people find themselves. But, as we shall see in the next chapter, parliamentarians' personal commitment to meditation practice and the democratisation of mental health are reflected in broader changes in governance structures in the UK. The social life of psychological knowledge links micro-level efforts of self-cultivation well beyond formal institutional structures with macro-level state agendas and governmental techniques. Mindfulness and mental health become transversal: patients, politicians, students, prisoners and others are understood to benefit from developing a universal capacity for awareness.

5

Mindful Politics, Participation and Evidence

AS WE HAVE SEEN in previous chapters, in recent years the category of mental health has expanded in Britain to include both those experiences that are associated with clinical diagnoses and the everyday stresses and strains of daily life. Patients, therapists and parliamentarians all experience themselves as affected by mental health, and they engage in dedicated practices to support their mental health both as a pragmatic preventative support and as a way of cultivating health and flourishing. Transformations in the category of mental health in Britain have shifted what is meant by the term, the people for whom it is a concern and the practices that are intended to address it. Mental health framed as 'something we all have' is neither a naturally occurring phenomenon nor a socially constructed fiction. As Eyal and colleagues write of comparable shifts in the categorisation of autism (Eyal et al. 2010, 30), '[t]he very structure of our knowledge—how we make distinctions—is what has changed'. In chapter 2 above I drew on Hacking's concept of 'looping' (Hacking 1995a; 1999; 2007) to account for the changing categorisation of depression and the development of secondary preventative interventions like MBCT. Certain human conditions are interactive, in that naming, classifying, diagnosing or treating them loops back and modifies the condition thus named. Such conditions often 'loop' because they become an identity, a way of relating to oneself or the motivation to work on oneself. They might also form the basis of people coming together and organising collectively in ways that give shape to their experiences. But distinctions between categorisations do not correspond to simple differences in the nature of things; categories are 'moving targets' (Hacking 2007) that shade into each other, requiring political deliberation, ethical and moral judgement, and economic calculation. As we saw in chapters 3 and 4 above, mental health is no longer framed as only affecting one in four people; rather, it is something we all have and something we can do something about. Mental health has become a transversal issue: state agents, intermediary representatives and those who are the target of state intervention are understood to share the cognitive fallibility that contributes to mental ill-health, *and* the capacity to improve their mental health by engaging in preventative practices.

This expands the focus of psychological governance from the treatment, regulation and control of specific individuals and populations to the cultivation of health for all people. Public mental health campaigns in Britain increasingly focus on primary prevention approaches that seek to stop mental health problems before they arise. Whereas tertiary prevention interventions aim to reduce the impact of ongoing illness, and secondary prevention strategies seek to prevent re-injury or recurrence of illness, primary prevention approaches are 'universal', in that they do not target populations specifically at risk but seek rather to benefit everyone. Scholars have framed mental health as a spectrum, stretching from 'mental disorder' to 'flourishing' (see Keyes 2002a; 2002b; see also Huppert 2005),[1] and have promoted primary prevention interventions as a way of supporting positive mental health in everyday life. Successive UK governments since the turn of the millennium have viewed the development of preventative, people-centred healthcare services as an approach by which the NHS might address the healthcare challenges of the twenty-first century, including ageing populations, high patient expectations and the evolving nature of disease (see, e.g., Department of Health 2008; 2009). Informed by academic research on positive mental health, psychological resilience and well-being, British national mental healthcare policy has identified the nurturance of human life as an aim of public health (see Huppert 2009; Layard 2005; Marks and Shah, 2005).

In this chapter, I focus on political interest in the policy potential of mindfulness. Parliamentarians who had completed the mindfulness course in Westminster set up an All-Party Parliamentary Group (APPG) to investigate the evidence and policy potential for mindfulness as a civil society intervention. APPGs are led by parliamentarians from different political parties who wish to cooperate on an area of policy or a specific issue for which there is cross-party interest (Norton 2008, 240). They are non-partisan groups, peripheral to the formal system of parliamentary decision-making, that rest on a collaboration between parliamentarians and non-parliamentary volunteers, and the majority of British APPGs are run on external support (see chapter 6 below).

While APPGs have existed in Westminster since the 1930s, they have prolifer-ated in recent years as informal cross-party fora in which dialogue between parliamentarians and 'stakeholders' can occur. Following the Labour Party election victory of 1997, the number of APPGs increased dramatically, with numbers more than doubling, from 242 to 592, by the time of the 2010 election. When the APPG on mindfulness began in 2014, there was a total of 609 APPGs in Westminster (Thomas 2014).

The Mindfulness APPG was launched at Westminster on 7 May 2014. Ap-proximately three hundred people crammed into the wood-panelled meeting room overlooking the Thames, including thirty MPs. In his presentation, Pro-fessor Willem Kuyken, a cognitive psychologist and the director of the Oxford Mindfulness Centre, described the meeting as 'a wow moment', and a sense of palpable excitement was in the air. The mission of the APPG was set out as being to provide a forum in parliament for discussion about the role of mind-fulness in public policy, promoting mindfulness for tackling a range of critical challenges that the government faced, advocating for more research to strengthen the existing evidence base and showcasing best practice.

Parliamentarians expressed their commitment to the Mindfulness APPG in both personal and political terms. In the press coverage around the launch, two of the parliamentary leads pointed to the mindfulness courses in parlia-ment (see chapter 4 above) as an impetus for the development of the APPG inquiry. Chris Ruane, the MP for the Vale of Clwyd, told the *Huffington Post* that in his view, 'the more we can develop mindfulness in the heart of parlia-ment and in the heart of government the more mindful policies we can de-velop' (Simons 2013). Similarly, in her interview on *Woman's Hour*, Tracey Crouch told the audience that politicians' own experiences of mindfulness informed the work of the APPG:

> What we are trying to do with the group is to apply some of the techniques that we have learnt as practitioners in parliament to policy development and to help other people, and it's certainly working very successfully in some parts of our public sector, whether it's education or the health service or even the criminal justice system, so I think that we are looking at how we can expand what we have learnt as practitioners into policy.

From May to December 2014, the APPG held eight hearings in Westminster to examine how mindfulness might benefit UK services and institutions. The scope of this inquiry was highly ambitious and brought together multiple policy areas and issues in diverse sectors of civil society in the UK. The eight parliamentary hearings were specifically targeted to address areas in which high levels of mental health diagnoses, stress or anxiety had been identified, coalescing under four broad headings: health, education, criminal justice and the workplace. They focused on, respectively, mindfulness in the workplace; mindfulness and mental health; mindfulness in the criminal justice system; mindfulness and physical pain; mindfulness for NHS staff; mindfulness in education; mindfulness in the workplace II; mindfulness and policing; and mindfulness and gangs. As a Labour MP emphasised at the launch, the aim of the inquiry was to 'gather the evidence for mindfulness and to present it in a non-party-political way so that those in power can look at the science of mindfulness and how it can help in our prisons, in our schools, in the health service and in the workplace'.

The Mindfulness APPG reflected wider trends in governmental culture, and the perception of a need for both evidence-based policy and participation in deliberative policy development by non-state actors. Public policy-making and governance in the UK have undergone significant changes in rationales and methods over the past two decades. Since the late 1990s, policy practice has increasingly emphasised evidence-based policy design focused on cost-effectiveness and 'what works', drawing on experts from outside politics to inform the development of policy objectives. Scientific evidence is increasingly incorporated into the political management and mitigation of risk. Over the same period, an emphasis on participatory governance has significantly influenced national and international political organisation.[2] The number of sites for producing and processing knowledge has proliferated, drawing on increasing amounts of citizen participation at the interface between science and politics. Knowledge is co-produced through the participatory deliberation of policy issues that are scientifically based, leading to new relationships among citizen/consumers, scientists and public administrators.

In what follows, I analyse the place of scientific evidence, personal testimony and meditation practice in the APPG. I argue that the APPG reflects the importance of evidence-based policy development and participatory governance in the UK more broadly. But I argue that the APPG on mindfulness was set apart from comparable participatory fora by the emphasis it placed on first-person experiences of mental health and mindfulness. Not only did members of the APPG hear scientific evidence and personal testimony on the benefits of mindfulness, but they also practised mindfulness themselves and understood their own experiences in terms of mental health and well-being. These first-person perspectives on mindfulness were a significant component of the APPG because of the broader transformations in the category of 'mental health' that I outlined above: mental health has expanded to include both disease categories and everyday struggles, and positive framings of mental health inform preventative interventions, simultaneously focused on the prevention of illness and the cultivation of health. While the co-production of deliberative politics rests on an increasing number of spaces for dialogue between the formal spaces of government and political subjects, in the participatory forum of the Mindfulness APPG both policy makers and citizens were addressed simultaneously as observers and as participants, engaging in the hearings as psychological and emotional subjects themselves.

The Scientisation of Politics and Participatory Governance

Since the 1990s the principle that health policy and practice should be based on systematically reviewed and critically appraised evidence of effectiveness (see Lambert 2005)[3] has increasingly informed political decision-making in what Maasen and Lieven refer to (2006, 400) as 'a *scientization of politics* and a *politicization of science*' (emphasis in original). Over the same period, in the wake of inadequate responses to unanticipated disasters (Jasanoff 1994; Petryna 2002), and rampant pandemics (Epstein 1996), activists and academics have argued that there are limits to purely technical forms of expertise and, furthermore, that experts and their advice are not neutral; that they are themselves embedded in techno-normative discourses (Nowotny 2003; see also Reardon 2007). Critics challenged what they identified as an absence of social concerns in technocratic governance and began to call for greater social accountability in policy-making (see Jasanoff 2003). While the framing of governance as the management of 'risk' remained significant (Beck 1992), risk discourse was challenged by the fact that the criteria for calculating risk were themselves deeply contested, and that radical uncertainty had become a condition of governance (Gottweis 2008, 280–81). Responding to complex issues required new modes of governance that could accommodate political distrust, a diversity of values and insecurity. In a response to the blurring of boundaries between science and politics, forms of participatory governance seemed to offer the promise of socially informed policy development, broadening deliberation about the values that inform policy, thereby increasing trust and subsequently more public support for policy outcomes. Thus, as evidence-based policy development has emerged, it has been met with calls for participatory forms of governance as an ethical redress to the perceived limits of 'technocratic' interventions. Under conditions of radical uncertainty, the language of ethics and morality emerged as a feature of governance (Bora and Hausendorf 2010, 2). Participatory governance offered a way of integrating normative principles and 'the values of society' into scientifically based policy development (Caduff 2010; Gottweis 2008).

The co-production of policies, based on increasing dialogue between the formal structures of the state and its subjects, requires an increasing involvement of non-state actors in spaces of government previously occupied by the formal state. As Pykett, Jones and Whitehead argue (2017, 1), '[t]here is now [. . .] a sense within the policy-making process that pragmatic, efficient and cost-effective policy change can and should be delivered through new forms of discursive fora and co-produced through participatory engagement with citizens'. Maasen and Lieven (2006) refer to these participatory settings as 'agoras': public spaces in which the political life of a city unfolds. Here, scientific knowledge is marshalled in the development of policy, and policy objects are shaped through the input of multiple contributors. These agoras rest on a recognition that expertise may be based on plural experiences that can be pooled in political problem solving through deliberative engagement. As Nowotny argues (2003, 153), '[b]y bringing in those previously excluded—at least symbolically—[. . .] the social distribution of expertise is recognised as instrumental in achieving good governance' (see also Shove and Rip, 2000). 'Expertise' is democratised and includes both 'experts' and 'stakeholders'. Maasen and Lieven put it thus (2006, 407–8):

> In this intermediary domain—neither purely scientific nor purely political—knowledge of various sources, as well as competing values and interests, can be discussed and negotiated. Here, political positions can be developed as a result of joint expertise and deliberatively produced policy recommendations.

In this way, they conclude (ibid., 408; emphasis in original), 'participatory settings (although with no direct influence) *resonate* in the political subsystem'.

Third- and Second-Person Perspectives: Evidence and Participatory Testimony

Each of the Mindfulness APPG hearings was fully attended, and I was told that it was unusual to have so many MPs present at APPG meetings, and even more unusual for them to stay for any length of time. Over the course of the inquiry,

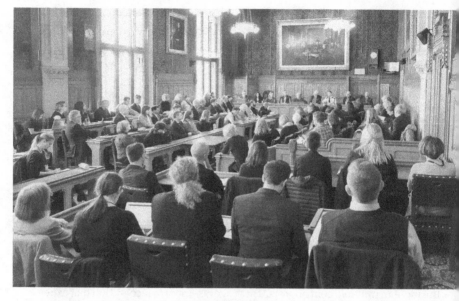

FIGURE 4. A meeting of the All-Party Parliamentary Group on Mindfulness, Westminster, October 2014. Photograph by Shai Dolev.

upward of eighty people presented statistics, scientific findings and accounts of professional practice and personal experience of mindfulness. Reflecting a commitment to evidence-based policy and the 'democratisation of expertise' (Liberatore and Funtowicz 2003), hearings incorporated evidence from service users and mental health workers, ex-offenders and probation officers, school children and educators, as well as researchers, NHS service commissioners and psychologists (see also Cook 2016). A volunteer advocate or a politician was responsible for chairing each of the meetings, which each followed a similar structure: a short introduction from one of the cross-party co-chairs acknowledging the extent to which parliamentarians had benefited from mindfulness courses in Westminster; a group mindfulness practice; presentation of statistics on the scale and economic implications of a particular societal problem; personal testimonials from people for whom mindfulness practice had been beneficial; an overview of the existing evidence base for mindfulness-based interventions; reports on the implementation of small-scale mindfulness interventions; discussion about the barriers to adoption of mindfulness in a given area; and an open discussion of coordination and next steps.

Throughout the inquiry process, research findings on mental health in different areas of civil society were collected together and presentations from scientific researchers made up a significant part of each of the hearings. As a Labour MP commented, the APPG was intended to 'support colleagues on all sides of the House and to make sure that the research that the scientists and professors do around the world doesn't lie gathering dust on shelves but is put into effective public policy for the reduction of misery in the world and the promotion of human flourishing'. Mental health issues were framed as sharing a common identity *and* as being unique to each domain. For example, at the hearing on criminal justice, statistics collected by the prison reform trust revealed that nearly half of the prison population suffers from depression or anxiety (Ministry of Justice 2013), and the suicide rate is almost fifteen times higher than in the general population (Department of Health 2005). At the hearing on mindfulness and the workplace, it was reported that since 2009 the number of sick days lost to stress, depression and anxiety has increased by 24 per cent (Mehta, Murphy and Lillford-Wildman 2014). Inquiry participants heard that in the next decade the cost of depression would rise to £9.19 billion a year in lost earnings alone, with an additional £2.96 billion in annual service costs (McCrone et al. 2008), that in England one in six adults met criteria for a common mental health problem such as anxiety or depression (McManus et al. 2014) and that one in eight of five–nineteen-year-olds met criteria for a mental health problem (NHS Digital 2018).

Clinical psychologists and neuroscientists presented the findings from systematic reviews, meta-analyses, randomised controlled trials and individual studies on mindfulness. For example, in the hearing on mindfulness and mental health, the audience heard that a meta-analysis of six randomised controlled trials found that MBCT reduced the risk of depressive relapse by almost half (43 per cent) in comparison to control groups for people who were currently well but who had had three or more depressive episodes (Piet and Hougaard 2011), that evidence suggests that MBCT reduces the severity of depressive symptoms in people currently experiencing an episode of depression (Strauss et al. 2014) and that a meta-analysis of studies in non-clinical populations suggested that MBSR can significantly reduce stress in comparison to control conditions (Chiesa and Serretti 2009). The hearing on physical pain heard that a review of 114 studies found consistent improvements in mental health and well-being (reductions in stress, anxiety and depression) in the context of poor physical health (Carlson 2012). In the hearing on mindfulness and education, the audience heard that recent meta-analyses of mindfulness-based initiatives (MBIs) for children and adolescents suggested improvements in stress, anxiety, depression and emotional and behavioural regulation, with larger effects reported in clinical than in non-clinical populations (Zoogman et al. 2015). In the hearing on the workplace, researchers reported that a number of randomised controlled trials of MBIs have found positive effects on burnout, well-being and stress (Mantos et al. 2014; Pidgeon, Ford and Klaassen 2014), and that mindfulness has been shown to improve higher cognitive skills, in relation to, for example, reaction times, comprehension scores, working memory functioning and decision-making (Mrazak et al. 2013; Zeidan et al. 2013). In the hearing on criminal justice, researchers emphasised that although studies were only indicative, they suggested that mindfulness improves self-regulation (Himelstein et al. 2012), reduces negative affectivity (Dafoe and Stermac 2013) and improves regulation of sexual arousal (Singh et al. 2011) and control of aggression (Singh et al. 2008). Altogether, however, through the orchestration of scientific evidence in the hearings, a troubling picture emerged, of a mental health epidemic in the UK. Econometric and psychological data on the projected costs, prevalence and severity of mental health problems and the evidence for mindfulness as a targeted intervention all pointed to an emerging public health crisis and the need for immediate funding, research and intervention to support vulnerable individuals and communities.

The third-person evidence of research was complemented by second-person accounts of personal and professional experience. I use 'second-person' here to refer to testimony presented in the APPG by expert witnesses. This is to differentiate it from first-person accounts of experience of mindfulness practice in the APPG, which I will go on to discuss below. Over the course of the eight hearings, various kinds of 'experts' provided evidence to the group. Representatives of the national government, members of the House of Lords, backbench politicians, scientists, regulators, professional healthcare workers, teachers, representatives of patient organisations, peer support workers and service users all contributed to the development of knowledge and political advice. At the APPG on Mindfulness and Mental Health, Helen, an MBCT participant who had been well and practising mindfulness for three years, spoke of her eleven-year history of treatment-resistant severe psychotic depression. She told the hearing that she had not been suicidal for three years and that she is now able to work. She described herself as a subversive mindfulness practitioner:

> I don't set a schedule but I practise for at least sixty minutes a day. I weave it into daily life when I need to and that's *often*. I've become adept at spotting changes in my mood, grounding, and calming down. I've become very very good at noticing.

Similarly, a woman called Helga told the group that she had participated in an MBCT course two years previously after suffering a long history of treatment resistant major recurrent clinical depression:

MBCT was a major breakthrough; within weeks a transformation started that continues now. But it's not for the faint hearted—to be with painful thoughts . . . not running away. It has affected my life as a whole and is a continuous ongoing process. I have never felt as alive as I do now.

In these personal testimonies, the value of mindfulness extended much further than it did in the research data. Mindfulness was presented as having had a profound and transformative effect on the speaker. For example, an ex-offender told the hearing on criminal justice of his previously troubled life, his discovery of mindfulness, and how much he had been affected by this. Preventing re-offence was implicit in his account, but he placed emphasis on his overall experience of life and his relationships with others:

I was diagnosed with PTSD [post-traumatic stress disorder] when I was five. My carers were violent. I didn't know what was happening. If you grow up in a war zone, you become a warrior. I got into alcohol and drugs. I ended up in prison. I had regret for the past and fear for the future. I was robbed of the present, and mindfulness gave that back. It's revolutionised my way of seeing the world and myself. My kids have never seen me violent and I'm trying to teach them through mindfulness. You have to try it. As they say in Glasgow, 'Better felt than telt.' I could tell you about all the miracles in my life, but you have to go out and taste it for yourself. Five years ago I was in a homeless shelter and now I'm sitting in parliament.

Testimonials were then followed by accounts from professionals who had introduced mindfulness-based interventions in their given field and the challenges that they had encountered. In the discussion about the challenges of implementing mindfulness, pragmatic issues such as funding and time were discussed as barriers in multiple areas. At the hearing on criminal justice, a senior representative for the Welsh probation service presented her experience of running a mindfulness pilot project in a probation hospital in Cardiff. This was conducted with two high-risk sexual offenders and one high-risk violent offender, all of whom had spent at least five years in prison. Simultaneously highlighting economic efficiency and personal transformation, she presented a case study of a violent offender who had used mindfulness to control his

impulse to commit a violent act. He had witnessed a young man being disre-
spectful to an older lady at a bus stop and was immediately awash with powerful fantasies of violence. He vividly imagined putting the young man's head
through the screen of the bus shelter, to the extent that he heard the glass
breaking and smelt the blood. At the same time, however, he heard his mindfulness teacher's voice in his head, saying, 'Notice what is happening right now.
Move towards the positive.' The probation executive told the hearing, 'He was
able to witness the thoughts in a non-judgemental way and allow them to pass
without reacting to them and being violent. We costed up that scenario and
found that it would have cost £100,000 in services if he had followed through
on that impulse.'

This combination of second- and third- person perspectives (testimonials
about experience and research findings) reflects new modes of governance
that emphasise citizen involvement in co-producing evidence-based policy. In
the hearing on mindfulness and mental health, clinical psychologists and an
NHS service commissioner gave expert witness, but so too did service users
from an NHS foundational trust. In the inquiry on mindfulness and criminal
justice, the audience heard testimony both from the head of public protection
from HMPPS (Her Majesty's Prison and Probation Service) in Wales and from
former offenders. And heads of educational trusts spoke on the same platform
as school children in the hearing on mindfulness and education. Inquiry hearings provided a site for participatory governance informed by a valorisation of
democratised expertise as significant for due process.

In the contemporary governmental emphasis on the democratisation of
expertise in participatory fora, the risk is that stakeholder testimony functions
as a moral alibi for political decisions (see Nowotny 2003), a feature of what
Jacob and Riles refer to (2007) as the 'new bureaucracies of virtue'. For example, Caduff demonstrates that the incorporation of participatory practices
into the development of public health policy in America built in an 'ethical
prophylaxis' to new policy on the distribution of influenza vaccinations (2010,
203; see also Franklin 2003). In the public engagement meetings developed to
deliberate pandemic influenza policy, responsibility for the facts and values
that informed deliberation fell to experts and the 'public' respectively. As
Caduff writes (2010, 208), '[i]n this model of public engagement scientific
experts are responsible for the determination of facts while ordinary citizens
are charged to deliberate about their normative implications'. The effort to
overcome the separation between facts and values—the aim that rendered

public participation in policy deliberation appropriate in the first place—was undercut by the demarcation of the roles of experts and publics. Participatory governance thus had the effect of generating a 'moral paper trail documenting the fact that ethical concerns have been taken into account in the making of public policy' (ibid., 214).

In the APPG, 'public' participation was actively constructed through the selection of presenters with shared forms of experience (see Caduff 2010; Gottweis 2008). What the school children, ex-offenders, NHS staff and former mental health patients had in common was stories of the ways in which their lives had been changed through mindfulness practice. Their testimonies of personal transformation complemented the thorough exploration of the third-person scientific evidence for mindfulness as a targeted intervention in specific populations. But the apportioning of responsibility for 'facts' and 'values' between 'experts' and 'publics' that Caduff identified in deliberation about vaccine policy was blurred in the APPG for two reasons. First, mental health was simultaneously framed in both negative and positive terms: as an epidemic that required action and as 'something we all have'. And second, mindfulness was framed both as a preventative intervention for those at risk of suffering from mental illness and as a practice that enabled people to live more fully. Mindfulness and mental health were cast as transversal issues, as personally relevant for politicians and cognitive psychologists as they were for service users and stakeholders.

'We're in This Together': First-Person Perspectives on Mental Health and Mindfulness

As we have seen, in the APPG expertise was democratised and authority rested on deliberation over multiple forms of evidence. As Nowotny writes of participatory fora (2003, 156), '[i]f we all are experts now, the order and ordering of the regime of pluralistic expertise will be played out and negotiated in this public space'. But what marked the APPG out from other participatory settings was that participants also engaged with third- and second-person perspectives on mental health from a first-person perspective. Mental health was presented as a transversal issue for everyone participating in the hearings. As Maasen and Lieven observe (2006, 408), in participatory settings, '[s]cientists, politicians, industrial actors and lay experts are addressed in two capacities: as experts *and* as citizens' (emphasis in original). As we have seen in earlier chapters, in the development of preventative healthcare interventions, mental health is democratised; the term refers simultaneously to those experiences that would constitute a diagnosis and the everyday ups and downs of daily life: as the category has expanded, it has come to encompass not just those who would qualify for a diagnosis, but all those who experience the setbacks and challenges, small or large, of life.[4] In so doing, mental health has shifted from an either/or state to a constituent component of life (we are all more or less well at different points in our lives) and prevention is framed in both negative and positive terms: it is concerned both with the prevention of ill-health and with the cultivation of positively valued mental health in daily life.

Mental health becomes something people can take care of in order to prevent mental illness and to encourage positive health. Introducing the APPG hearing on mental health, the chair commented to the room, 'You're all experts, as it were. We're all really peers in this.' Mental health was understood to be 'something we all have' and learning to relate to the mind in a healthy way was described as a constitutive component of living well. Addressing the hearing on mindfulness in the workplace, a university professor specialising in the psychology of organisations described the value of non-judgemental awareness 'for everyone from the front-line porter to the secretary of state'. As he said to the audience,

> As a result of sitting [in meditation] I become more aware of experience. So many thoughts going round in our heads, 'Is my tie straight?' 'Do I seem nervous?' 'Are they going to make a judgement about me?' These thoughts are the social conditioning that we respond to and that distracts us from immediate experience of the moment.

As Gottweis writes of participatory deliberation (2008, 281), 'in moralized or ethicized issue areas, people take the first-person stance on issues; they raise and discuss questions such as: "What are *we* supposed to do?", "What shall *we* do next?", "What is the right thing for *me*/for *us* to do?"' (emphasis in original). In the APPG, people from diverse walks of life related the issues of mindfulness and mental health to themselves and their own actions, and thus took on a participant's *as well as* an observer's point of view.

Mindfulness and mental health were framed as transversally relevant. At the start of each hearing, assembled participants settled into a short mindfulness practice led by a respected mindfulness teacher. As one of the parliamentary co-chairs commented at the hearing on mindfulness and mental health, this short practice was important, because we were there to discuss mindfulness, and this ought to be done mindfully. Wooden benches creaked and papers rustled as, with very little prompting, assembled parliamentarians, scientists and citizens adjusted their postures in preparation for the practice, moving further back into the chairs, straightening their backs and settling into meditation. All around the room, politicians, healthcare workers, and service users fell silent and sat upright, devices and notes put down so that their hands could rest in their laps. As a clinical psychologist took the microphone to lead the short practice in this hearing, he commented, 'Gosh, just look around the room. Everyone's shifting their posture and finding an anchor.' He guided participants to close their eyes or lower their gaze: 'Bringing your attention voluntarily, with intention, with care, with wisdom, with patience, with curiosity, maybe to the breath in the belly. Through the full duration of this in-breath . . . and this out-breath . . . this in-breath . . . this out-breath . . . there it is.'

Mindfulness practices were usually only a few minutes long, but had the effect of shifting the feeling of the room. The excitement of arrival and the bustle of finding seats, saying hellos and scanning the room to see who was there gave way to a focused sense of engagement. Thanking the meditation teacher in the APPG on criminal justice, the parliamentary chair described the value of mindfulness practice in both personal and political terms. She told the room, 'I have a small chart next to my desk, in which I mark my emotional experience, like an emotional barometer, and I've found myself going from a siege mentality to periods of inexplicable happiness.' As she spoke, her words were received by nodding around the room. 'I can see that I don't have to sell it to you,' she remarked, and assured the meeting that

> the expert evidence that we're pooling here will set us up as members of parliament to present a positive case to our ministers, whatever party they are from. This is an idea whose time has come. Because it's practical, because it works, because you can see the results, you can feel the results.

Reflecting the presentation of his cross-party colleague, a Labour MP told the audience that 'we've developed our personal practice and we're now looking to bring this into policy practice on a non-party political basis taking on board the evidence here today'.

Politicians' personal meditation practice informed the ways in which they deliberated about mindfulness in the APPG. Participation was premised on a recognition of the centrality of feeling and emotion in public sector work. As Whitehead et al. state (2017, 196), 'changing the ways in which government relates to people's behaviours has significant implications for how we understand the subject position of civil servants themselves'. The former Conservative Party co-chair of the APPG, Tracy Crouch, told one meeting,

> Those of you at the front can see that I am barefoot; why might this be? Because mindfulness taught me how to anchor myself through my feet. And you might think that it is rare for a politician, but I hate public speaking. Inside right now, I am a jittery wreck. I find that being barefoot helps me, in terms of calming myself, creating the right posture, and delivering a speech in the House of Commons.

She went on to tell the hearing that she welcomes mental health as part of the conversation in parliament:

> How it doesn't always matter if you're not always the strongest cookie. How sometimes its okay to recognise your strengths and your weaknesses as one thing. And I think I'm really pleased that mindfulness has now become something that we talk about as politicians and how we deal with all the pressures that we face, and how we can spread that across the world.

This universal framing of mental health as 'something we all have' informs a recognition of the centrality of feeling and emotion in public sector work, and the idea that '[p]olicy makers themselves are of course subject to the same cognitive biases and impulses as citizens' (Pykett et al. 2016, 78). In what Gottweis refers to (2008, 281) as the 'ethicization and emotionalization of governance', parliamentarians were recognised as psychological subjects themselves. Writing twenty years ago, Nikolas Rose identified the formation of modern psychological enterprise in England as focused on the abnormal functioning of individuals (1989; 1998; see also 2010, 96), leading to policies targeted towards 'risky' individuals or groups that are deemed guilty of regularly making poor decisions. Today, the reframing of mental health as a transversal issue means that politicians are understood to be susceptible to the same mooded biases and problematic thinking patterns as the populations that are the targets of policies.

It was this transversal understanding of the category of mental health that informed the APPG hearings: mental health affects politicians, prisoners and nurses alike, and all people could benefit from learning how to take care of their own mental health in response to the mounting pressure of modernity. For example, at the second hearing, on mindfulness and health, an A&E (Accident and Emergency) mental health nurse who works nights and has two teenage sons reported to the hearing that she joined a mindfulness course at work out of curiosity and that it had had a radical impact on her life:

> It's been quite life-changing for me. I found quite quickly that my thought processes changed and I hadn't realised that maybe I had got quite bogged down in things; I just thought it was the passage of life and it takes its toll on everyone. You know, we all have bereavements, we all have losses, things go wrong in our lives. During the course, I was just like my old self, just like when I was a lot younger. I was happy, I was feeling joy in things, and I hadn't realised that that part of my life had gone.

This transversal relevance of good mental health for service users and health-care professionals was reflected in the hearing on mindfulness and education, during which both teachers and schoolchildren spoke about their mindfulness practice. Speakers highlighted the problems of retaining staff because of the stress of teaching, the statistics on children's mental health and the evidence for mindfulness as a preventative intervention and as a support for non-academic skills and capabilities, such as 'character building' and 'resilience' (see chapter 6 below). Similarly, in the hearing on criminal justice, speakers presented mindfulness as relevant to prison officers and prisoners alike. As an officer from a charity trust providing mindfulness in prisons told the hearing,

> What can be vital is working with staff. So not only working with prisoners but with staff. To teach officers first or alongside prisoners so that they would be able to encourage students/prisoners to come in because they know the benefits in managing their wings and use them as facilitators.[5]

As the mental health charity Mind has stated (Mind 2017), now, 'mental health is everyone's business'.

Conclusion: Transversal Mental Health and Participatory Politics

In this chapter I have examined the relationship between the category of mental health and public and political interest in mindfulness through an eth-nographic focus on the UK parliamentary mindfulness APPG. What emerges is that transformations in participatory governance and preventative health-care become mutually implicating: deliberation over the policy potential for mindfulness in the UK reflects broader changes in understandings of mental health and human flourishing, and these changes informed the participatory forum of the APPG. Through a combination of first-, second- and third-person evidence, mindfulness was deliberated over as a universally relevant, psychologically informed, practice. The third-person perspective of scientific findings provided persuasive representations of the character and scale of the challenges in each policy area, and of the evidence base for mindfulness. The second-person accounts of personal testimonials and professional reports provided impactful descriptions of experience for attendees. These resonated with the first-person experience of mindfulness practice that began each hearing and the universalist framing of mental health that involved attendees as simultaneously observers and as participants.

In a totally utilitarian reading, interest in preventative mental healthcare may be seen as an effort to avoid the burden on Britain's NHS of chronic mental ill-health. An emphasis on the prevention of illness and the cultivation of health often requires the modification of quotidian 'healthy behaviour'. For example, those who suffer from physical conditions such as heart disease, diabetes and some forms of cancer are encouraged to manage mundane behaviours in order to reduce the impact of ongoing illness. In such approaches, emphasis is placed on empowering people to make better decisions for themselves and change their behaviour in ways that improve long-term health outcomes, which will lead to improvements in health overall at the levels of both the individual and the population as a whole.[6] This creates an impetus for action, a biopolitical case for disciplining and regulating healthy populations. And yet, engagement with preventative mental healthcare (and healthcare more generally) is hard to capture in narrow consequentialist parameters. The category of mental health extends into the relationship that a person has with herself and the choices that she makes about her lifestyle and behaviour, and it includes the subjective values and shared beliefs that motivate or inhibit health-seeking behaviours. Calls for primary prevention interventions are not just the site for a 'realist' or functionalist mental healthcare that will help people to manage emotions and reduce stress. They are also informed by a positive idea that through the cultivation of mental health, everyday life might emerge as the site for flourishing and well-being.

In preventative healthcare, the locus of intervention often lies far outside the remit of medical science and encompasses the relationship an individual has with herself, and the subjective values and shared beliefs that motivate or inhibit health-seeking behaviours. The categorisation of mental health as 'something we all have', and the introduction of mindfulness as a way of supporting positive mental health, neutralise or sidestep the antinomies of medicalisation—between health and illness, between normal life and pathology, between living well and preventing symptoms and between expert and patient. While acute depression might be treated with antidepressant medication, an emphasis on the cultivation of positive mental health is not limited to a strictly medical domain. On the basis of a positive representation of health as well as the prevention of illness, mental health is conceived of as spectrum experience that can be tended to and cultivated rather than an illness that can be cured or a disease that can be removed; living well is associated with cultivating good mental health for all people. Thus, mental health, through a series of looping processes, comes to cover a wider and wider spectrum, becoming a universal constituent of modern life.

In her ethnography of the rapid expansion of mental healthcare in Nepal following the 2015 earthquake, Chase calls (2019) for anthropological analyses to work with, rather than against, the vagaries of the category of 'mental health', arguing that the term retains different meanings in different places, and that this enables psychosocial global mental health services to be 'scaled up', pointing to the relationship between how we think about suffering and the way we attend to it. In the UK, emphasis on prevention and the characterisation of mental health as a transversal issue determines what we think we can legitimately do about it, 'reshaping our notions of self and ways of being' (Kirmayer 2015b, 525). 'Mental health' becomes personally relevant for both experts and patients (we all have mental health) in both the cultivation of health and the prevention of illness (we are all more, or less, well at any given time). This understanding of the nature of the mind as susceptible to patterns of emotional reactivity and attentional 'hijacking' informs state and non-state actors' perceptions of the value of and need for psychology-based policies; and the sense of horizontal fraternalism that this generates is reflected in stakeholder involvement, participatory governance and collaboration in new approaches to governance. In contrast to the separation of facts and values identified by Caduff (2010), participation in the APPG at Westminster was informed by a sense of democratic and existential inclusivity. It rested on a decentred understanding of governance that emphasised practices of 'co-production' through the orchestration of state and non-state actors, and an underlying universalist and ethicised rationale for dialogue and collaboration.

As we have seen, the pragmatism of practitioners' engagement with mindfulness practices as they seek to support their mental health is complemented by a Romantic aspiration to 'live fully'. In the APPG, mindfulness was presented as both rational and ethical; it was both shown to 'work' in the pragmatic and targeted reduction of mental ill-health, and to be a personally transformative practice in the positive framing of mental health as a constituent component of flourishing; and the case for it was made both through statistical and scientific evidence and through an emphasis on participatory deliberation and experience. It is to the ongoing tension between ethical and economic value that I turn next.

6

The Skilful Means of the
Mindful Advocate

[A] way of being in wise and purposeful relationship with one's experience.

—JON KABAT-ZINN, 'FOREWORD', *MINDFUL NATION UK*

But does it work?

—NHS SERVICE COMMISSIONER, 2015

IN 2015, the *Mindful Nation UK* report (MAPPG 2015a) was launched in Westminster, marking the culmination of the APPG inquiry process we examined in the last chapter. The report cited research that points to an ongoing mental health crisis in Britain, outlining the character and scale of challenges identified in health, education, the workplace and the criminal justice system, and the existing evidence for the efficacy of mindfulness-based interventions. It did this by setting out the economic case for preventative mental health support, calling for targeted interventions in each area and funding for further research. As a complement to this, each section of the report contained two to four pages of case studies from people who had benefited from mindfulness. These were written in the first-person and were personal stories of the lived impact of mindfulness practice. In short, the efficient collation of econometric and statistical research findings and qualitative accounts in the report presented a troubling picture of a costly mental health crisis, beginning in the health sector and extending through the education system, the criminal justice system and the workplace. The report identified and costed problems in society, highlighted policy objectives and made a case for mindfulness as a scientifically appropriate and economically responsible solution. In effect, mindfulness was presented as both instrumental (it could be used) and goal-orientated (it would work).

While the report went on to influence political policy (see below) and, to date, has been downloaded over thirty thousand times, it also attracted criticism. For example, it was criticised by two reviewers for promoting mindfulness as 'a method that "works"' (Moloney 2016, 283) in the service of 'specific operational objectives' (Hyland 2016, 134). Hyland argues (ibid., 134–35) that the 'transformational function' of mindfulness has been 'co-opted in order to achieve specific *operational* objectives, and such pragmatic purposes have obscured the links with the foundational moral principles' (emphasis in original) as mindfulness has 'swept virus-like through academia, public life and popular culture' (ibid., 133). Similarly, Moloney thinks (2016, 270) that mindfulness is 'at the forefront of an official utilitarian "mental health" movement, sweeping through the health and social sciences'. He describes the report as blending 'a declared humanitarian commitment with a strong fiscal case for psychological treatment (in this case, "mindfulness") as a means of reducing healthcare bills through the prevention of psychological distress, and by getting the disturbed and disabled back to work and off the state sickness benefits roster' (ibid., 271), and he argues that 'mindfulness could never be a treatment or method that "works" in a relatively straightforward way, like swallowing a medicinal pill' (ibid., 283).

The report had been written by a group of unpaid non-political advocates over an eight-month period following the inquiry process. No one in this group had any previous experience of political advocacy, and each member was motivated to participate by their personal commitment to mindfulness. In this chapter, I focus on how the *Mindful Nation* report was drafted in order to provide an ethnographic account of advocacy in an era of evidence-based policy-making. Analysis of the report divorced from the social processes through which it was created and to which it contributes would risk presenting mindfulness as an instrumentalised tool of governance. But an abstract denunciation (or celebration, for that matter) of 'instrumentalisation' and 'evidence' makes little sense in anthropological terms, because the mere fact of instrumentalisation tells us very little about the causes and effects of practices of governance in any given context (see du Gay 2005). Like many others, I am cautious of the effects of instrumentalisation and the utilitarian logics of audit and accountancy measures (see for example Hoggett 2005; Miller 2005), and yet, dwelling on the reduction of ethical practices to an instrumentalist agenda misses the opportunity to explore the ways in which such agendas are developed and the creative effects that they generate. What can an ethnographic account of political advocacy reveal about explanatory practices? What kinds of case are compelling? What makes an explanation persuasive? And how is this achieved?

Volunteers became political advocates because they believed that mindfulness is a personally transformative practice and that it is foundational for living well. At the same time, in order to make mindfulness intelligible as a policy object, it had to be framed in utilitarian and economic terms. With an analytical focus on the social practices of advocacy, I examine how volunteer advocates resolved the (potentially) uncomfortable relationship between the ethical value that mindfulness held for them and their use of governmental technologies, political discourses and economic rationales. The relationship between the ethopoetic processes associated with self-cultivation and broader economic and political logics raises significant ethnographic questions about the negotiation and coordination of different kinds of knowledge, values and interests. How do political advocates negotiate conflicting values? How do they integrate their motivating values with their knowledge about action? And what do they think of as being the right way to coordinate in order to reach their goal? In what follows, I unpack the practices of knowledge management by which the policy potential of mindfulness was made persuasive, and I show that in the process of drafting the *Mindful Nation* report, volunteer advocates learned to navigate political technologies and discourses and to negotiate a balance between ethical and economic values.

In a series of papers, Michael Lambek makes a persuasive case for maintaining a clear analytical distinction between the meanings of 'value' in ethical and in economic practice and cautions against conflating the two (see also Tambiah 1990, 150).[1] Ethical and economic values are incommensurable because they are constituted in clearly distinct ways and there are points at which they simply do not meet; they are 'isomorphous and each leaves a remainder' (Lambek 2008b, 139). For Lambek (2008b), ethical value is characterised by the exercise of judgement in ongoing personal practice, and is contingent on context and multiple considerations. Liberal economic value, by contrast (Lambek 2008a), is characterised by its 'utility' and informs concepts arising from abstract reasoning, economic rationalisation and bureaucratic justification (ibid., 310). Ethical values are absolute and incommensurable, expressed as practices of judgement, while economic values are relative and commensurable.[2]

Lambek's distinction helpfully puts a finger on an ethnographic puzzle at the heart of *Mindful Nation*. Utility theories of value do not account for the experience, value and effect of learning to relate to oneself mindfully that motivated volunteer advocates to write the report. Volunteers described mindfulness as 'a way of being', and their passion for mindfulness has a clear affinity with Lambek's conception of moral judgement and ethical value, because it gave them what he might refer to as 'the practical means to engage ethically with the present and to anticipate the future by means of practices established and dispositions cultivated in the past' (2008a, 125). At the same time, however, political advocacy is in itself *necessarily* instrumentalising; it is an effort to effect change in the world, however that change might be conceived. Furthermore, the presentation of mindfulness in the report and the evidence gathered for its efficacy were clearly informed by a utility theory of value. To put it at its simplest, it is unlikely that mindfulness would be being discussed in parliament as a 'way of being' if it were not for the development of an evidence base for its efficacy. In order to ask, 'Does it work?', means and ends must be separated, and ends must be framed as measurable objects, rather than as qualities of acts (virtue) or of actors (character) (Lambek 2008b, 136).

In what follows, I examine the explanatory requirements attached to making a case for mindfulness in a policy context. I ask by what means such a case is produced, and whom it serves; how authority is constructed in political advocacy, and through what technologies it is made persuasive; and how people relate political practices to understandings of ethical life. This chapter is inspired, in part, by a Foucauldian concern with the relationship between forms of political rationality and specific technologies of government, as encapsulated in Foucault's theory of governmentality. But whereas governmentality is seen by some (e.g., Shore and Wright 2000) as purely an instrument of coercion, I argue that engagement with technologies of government opens up new spaces of reflection and political negotiation (see Born 2002). Thus, this chapter illustrates the simple point that explanatory practices may be constituted by multiple, and sometimes competing, types of value. I focus on the interrelationship between personal ethics, normative imperatives and new technologies of government in order to explore the processes of knowledge management that are central to bureaucratic practice and political advocacy. Over the eight months that it took to arrive at the *Mindful Nation* report in its final form, volunteer advocates learned to navigate political technologies in order to be 'heard'; that is, to shape mindfulness as a credible policy object. This recursivity, explaining mindfulness and in the process transforming it, suggests that policy development and advocacy are non-linear processes, and that they are informed as much by ethical and normative as by epistemological or economic agendas.

Learning Advocacy and Drafting the Report

The volunteer advocates who wrote the *Mindful Nation* report were brought together by their enthusiasm for mindfulness. They constituted a group of highly professionalised people, including a senior journalist, senior academics, the chief operating officer for an educational trust, the clinical lead for an NHS trust, a director of the Royal Society of Arts, a director from the corporate sector, a chief executive from the probation service, clinical psychologists and others. Each of them had experience of mindfulness in their respective professional worlds and all had a committed personal meditation practice, in some cases extending back for decades, but none of them had been involved in political advocacy before. Political advocacy and the APPG were thrilling. Volunteers were excited that the APPG and drafting of the report were powered by a groundswell of 'grass roots' support by passionate independent practitioners.

Immediately after the eighteen-month APPG inquiry process, the volunteers drafted a twelve-page interim report (MAPPG, 2015b), which was launched in parliament a month later to muted applause. This report summarised the findings of the inquiry process and referred to the considerable popularity of mindfulness in the UK, citing widespread media coverage, high demand for mindfulness courses and the popularity of books and CDs that draw on mindfulness-based interventions. In all, the brief document provided information on the outcomes of the hearings, but few references to research on mindfulness. And while it referenced concerns about the economic cost of a mental health crisis, it placed emphasis on the possibilities of 'transformation' and 'wisdom' that the volunteers believed arose through mindfulness practice. As they wrote (MAPPG 2015b, 1)

> We find that mindfulness is a transformative practice, leading to a deeper understanding of how to respond to situations wisely. We believe that government should widen access to mindfulness training in key public services, where it has the potential to be an effective low-cost intervention with a wide range of benefits.

The parliamentarians were not happy, and summoned representatives of the volunteers to parliament for a meeting. The volunteers reported back to the group that they had (figuratively) had their wrists slapped: The interim report simply did not work as an advocacy document. The parliamentarians wanted to see evidence of the scales and costs of the problems to be addressed, the evidence for the appropriacy of mindfulness-based interventions in each case, and for all of this information to be embedded in established political discourse. In addition to relating it to the policy challenges presented by mental health, mindfulness needed to be framed in terms of alternative metrics such as well-being and resilience. That is, problems and their potential solutions had to be identified, backed by evidence, and costed, and mindfulness had to be couched in terms of existing political and economic narratives. As Susan, a senior journalist, told me,

> They were applying a very New Labour policy framework to it. Everything that we do in terms of social spending has to be absolutely bottomed out in terms of its impact, value for money: 'This is how much you spend, this is how much you save.'

The parliamentarians' feedback on the interim report reflects a dominant strand of contemporary governmental culture. As we saw in the last chapter, in an era of evidence-based policy-making, governmental agendas increasingly rest on evidence for efficacy and accountability. In the later decades of the twentieth century, political decision-making became increasingly dependent on scientific knowledge and experts, reflecting the assumption that the empirical tools of randomised controlled trials (RCTs), advanced statistical analysis and social science could improve public policy. Explanatory cases for policy development increasingly rested on scientific evidence for 'what works' (Davies, Nutley and Smith 2000), and health policy and practice (and indeed other areas of social policy) came increasingly to be based on systematically reviewed and critically appraised evidence of effectiveness.

The volunteer advocates felt deeply frustrated by the parliamentarians' response. They had intended the interim report to act as a placeholder while they began the big job of drafting the final report. But the comments from the parliamentarians raised important questions about what ought to go into the report and what it was for. What kind of explanation of mindfulness would be persuasive? And could it be presented as an evidence-based technique without detracting from the value that it held for the volunteers? Volunteer advocates felt that, while they clearly *could* make an evidence-supported and economic case for mindfulness, such utilitarian terms were ill-suited to explaining its ethical value. They felt strongly that econometric justification needed to be

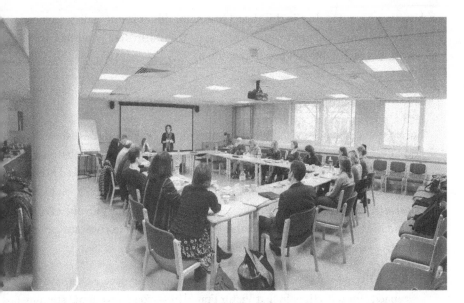

FIGURE 5. Drafting the report of the All-Party Parliamentary Group on
Mindfulness, London, December 2017. Photograph by author.

balanced by a representation of mindfulness as an ethical practice with the
potential to transform society. Thus the challenge of the writing process for
the volunteers became to produce an account that struck a balance between
the ethical value of reflective self-awareness and the economic value of pragmatic and measurable outcomes.

On the day of the first drafting meeting, I walked to the sandwich shop with
Danny, an NHS senior executive, and I asked him what he thought success
would look like: what would it mean to live in a 'mindful nation'? Danny had
been practising meditation for thirteen years. He first came across mindfulness while he was doing a CBT training course and started practising mindfulness while he was on his commute to work. He told me that for him, a
mindful nation would be 'a society that is more awake, compassionate, more
interested in processes than results'. Returning to the meeting with our sand-
wiches, though, he told me that if the report was going to have any political
impact it would need to make targeted recommendations with specific outcomes that were economically and statistically justified. Recommencing the
drafting process after lunch, he said to the group, 'As a health professional, I'm
a secularised philosopher in a way, and we're asking the question, "What is a
good life? How do we lead a good life?"' Reflecting on the challenge ahead,

however, he noted that 'in this thrust to get mindfulness into policy, we need to do it pragmatically but without losing its transformative potential. That's why this is such a difficult one to pin down.'

Personal Ethics vs. Political Evidence

For volunteer advocates, the value of mindfulness lay in both the experience and effect of developing a relationship with one's own mind: a relationship that they thought resulted from meditation practice. Tom, who worked in education and had been practising meditation for twenty years, was keen to emphasise this in our discussions over the writing period. In the pub one evening he told me that, for him, the real value of mindfulness lay in cultivating metacognitive awareness:

> It feels like what it's seeking to create is metacognitive space, isn't it, and that capacity for reflection. In that Victor Frankl bit—you know, about stimulus and response and the gap, and the gap is our power to choose, and in that power to choose is our growth and our freedom. It feels like that capacity for metacognition is the name of the game. It's the name of the game.[3]

In Tom's view, people might learn to relate to themselves with mindful awareness, and this was of value, because it led to the freedom to discern a wise response to experience. Others shared this view. They thought that having an ongoing mindful relationship with themselves was valuable, not as a goal of practice but for its own sake. As Danny told me when we met up for tea in the British Library,

> I think mindfulness connects us to being human, and being part of the species *sapiens sapiens*. It's sad that we're all going to get old and ill and die, and it requires a huge amount of compassion. And we all have to somehow support each other and be in a community that supports us with that existential reality.

For Danny and others, learning to relate to oneself and others with mindful awareness was an important motivator in their voluntary work. For Sarah, a cognitive psychologist who had been practising mindfulness for twenty-five years, for example, this pointed to a possible societal sea-change, if mindfulness were widely practised:

> The thing that's really lighting me up at the moment is the potential for this work to stimulate systemic change and the sense that the human mind is at

the basis of everything we do. And if we can, as a society, really get skilful about how we think about and use and cultivate our minds, well, that's going to have an impact across all sectors. So, it's something about just really being explicit on a societal level that this is important and that it's not just about mindfulness as a tool, but mindfulness is one tool that can support skilful use of the human mind.

Sarah was motivated to volunteer her time by personal conviction and a sense of shared ethical feeling with other advocates. Similarly, Adam Reed has highlighted the relationship between private moral enthusiasm and an ethics of professionalism in his ethnography of a Scottish animal protection charity (Reed 2017a; 2017b). He demonstrates that participation in the charity is based on a convergence of private and organisational values, and the success of the charity is thought to rest on the moral enthusiasm of its staff (2017a). Mindfulness advocates were motivated by their personal meditation practice and their professional experience. This drove enormous commitment to the advocacy process, which was at times in tension with the work of advocacy itself.

For many of the volunteers, instrumental explanations of the effects of mindfulness did not capture why it was important to them. For example, the idea that living well might be understood in instrumental terms did not sit well with Teresa, a mental health professional. As she told me,

If we were just farm animals, it would be fine. A lot of NICE[4] guidance for later life is like that. Look after the 'old person animal'. Exercise, nutrition, warmth. But the things that make people live independently, have quality of life and look after themselves are feeling valued, feeling they've got something to give, to get up for—all those things that are about us as feeling human beings with a sense of self, identity or purpose'.

After a meditation practice at the beginning of a drafting meeting, she turned to me and asked, 'really, how are you going to measure this?' Furthermore, volunteers thought that the tension they felt between ethical and economic values was reflected in parliamentarians' engagement with mindfulness as well. As Sarah told me in a formal interview during the drafting process,

There's something really interesting about that whole parliament thing. It's almost as if there were two parallel things happening for those politicians. The reason I think that some of them really got behind this was because of their own personal mindfulness practice. That awakened something in them. You'd need to inquire with them, but I suspect it was something about reconnecting to personal values, personal meaning, a sense of sanity about how we can live our lives. So there's that element, but alongside that there's this other element which they have to buy into about policy development and looking at mindfulness in a much more instrumental way, about the sorts of things that policy makers have to talk about like cost-effectiveness and productivity and presenteeism and efficiency and use of attentional resources. So, they're both true, but I think there's potentially a hazard with majoring on the instrumental aspect of it. Because actually that's not what's going to sustain the reasons for practicing this.

This relationship between ethical commitment and evidence was reflected in the development of the report as volunteer advocates navigated what they saw as the ill fit between the 'intangible', ethical nature of mindfulness and the standard categories used to identify policy areas and the measures used to assess outcomes.

Political Narratives

In a document circulated to the group, the head of a national charity provided volunteers with advice about how to think about their work. In developing the report, they were encouraged to think carefully about *why* mindfulness *might* be a policy issue. For example, were there specific policy 'asks': two or three specific areas in which they hoped to make an impact? Volunteers were asked to consider how these might fit into a devolved system environment, in which executive control is increasingly local or regional. The document suggested that 'rather than generating interest that isn't already there', they should 'find conversations that are already going on and be part of them [and] be part of existing conversations around mental health, wellbeing economics or procedural fairness in criminal justice, for example'. Articulating mindfulness in relation to broader political narratives became a central focus of the eight-month writing period. As anthropologist Maia Green argues of her work as a development policy analyst and advisor, in order to explain why policy objectives should receive funding, development categories have to be reordered and worked out so that they can become 'thinkable, malleable and ultimately real' (Green 2011, 41). Quite consciously, mindfulness was incorporated into political narratives focused in different ways on the mind, which were supported by alternative metrics. Volunteers worked to explain mindfulness in terms of emerging political narratives about mental health, character, attention, happiness, well-being and resilience. Each of these 'buzzwords' referenced wider social interests at the time and offered a way of embedding mindfulness in conversations that were already taking place. Drafting the report involved researching these conversations, marshalling scientific evidence on mindfulness and establishing a relationship between the two.

Such narrative framings were not a fabrication of the advocates—these were already widespread in academic and political literature. For example, 'well-being' has emerged as a key economic and development focus (see Clark 2002; Crisp and Hooker 2000; Dasgupta 1993; 2001; Griffin 1986; Sen 1999). It was incorporated into the United Nations Development Index, and informed the development of the metrics of quality- and disability-adjusted life years by the World Health Organization (WHO) (Cummins 2005). Well-being has comfortably become a standard narrative and metric in political models of prosperity and development. As a political narrative, well-being enables the marriage of wide-ranging ideas about health, education, opportunity, empowerment and capability with broader metrics such as affluence, gender or the environment. Linked to this are broader issues of 'quality of life' (Nussbaum and Sen 1993; Offer 1996), leading some to describe 'well-being' and 'quality of life' as a 'global morality dictum' (Strathern 2005). Similarly, 'resilience' became a part of mainstream development language in Britain after it was placed 'at the heart' of the UK government's 'Humanitarian Emergency Response Review' in 2011 (Ashdown 2011, 4). The term 'resilience' was developed in the physical sciences to describe the qualities and capacities that enable a community to recover from a catastrophic event (Barrios 2016), focusing on the mechanisms that enable a system to return to equilibrium after a stress or the ability to absorb change (Gordon 1978; Holling 1973, 14). 'Resilience' soon extended from political interest in infrastructure to a focus on human capacity, however, becoming a core part of DFID (Department for International Development) work and education policy. Political focus on psychological vulnerability is informed by concerns about mental health. Here, 'resilience' indicates psychological characteristics that enable individuals to 'bounce back' from challenging circumstances and to weather the everyday stresses of life (Ryff et al. 1998).

The value of mindfulness could easily be explained in the language of 'well-being' or 'resilience'. Psychological research suggests that mindfulness practice plays a role in psychological well-being (e.g., Brown and Ryan 2003; Josefsson et al. 2011). Attention and impulse control have been linked to social well-being indicators as wide-ranging as criminal record, addiction, ability to maintain committed relationships and body mass index (see Moffitt et al. 2011). And mindfulness is believed to help those who practise it to cope with life (from stress, anxiety and depression to impulse control, emotional regulation and intellectual flexibility) through the cultivation of psychological resilience (see, e.g., Bajaj and Pande 2016; Shapiro, Brown and Biegel 2007). If earlier models of resilience were characterised by a resilient subject who withstood or overcame oppressive conditions through their inner capacities for survival, 'post-classical' models of resilience frame the resilient subject as thriving in an interactive process of relational adaption. In response to intractable and complex policy problems, resilience takes the form of 'an emergent and adaptive process of subject/object interrelations' (Chandler 2014, 7) requiring self-reflexivity and relational sensitivity (ibid., 9).

As a political narrative for mindfulness, 'well-being' had many advantages. Well-being had formed the basis of previous policy work that had led to important changes in the provision of mental health services and training in the UK and had been treated as an object of empirical knowledge informed by value judgements about the good life (Alexandrova 2017). But as a narrative, well-being was also felt to come with its own challenges. The multifaceted nature of well-being makes it a useful tool in qualitative research but made it hard for the volunteer advocates to develop a clear workable presentation of its value, its measurement and its outcomes in relation to mindfulness as a narrative bed for advocacy. For example, in Shadow Cabinet discussions about mindfulness in the run-up to the 2015 election it was anticipated that a framework of well-being might be critiqued as too 'fluffy' by opponents on both the right and the left, and that it did not present an economically credible focus for investment. On 7 May, a general election saw the Conservative Party gain an outright majority, unshackling the Conservative government from its unpopular coalition with the Liberal Democrats and confounding the predictions of opinion polls and political analysts alike. In their manifestos, each of the political parties had made strong commitments to increased provision for mental health, and the Labour Party had gone further, in promising that mental health would be given the same priority as physical health. In Labour's manifesto, the party hedged their narrative bets by pledging to introduce mindfulness as a support for young people's well-being *and* resilience (Labour Party 2015, 35).

Volunteers were able to draw on this existing language to explain the value of mindfulness for parliamentarians, and they were confident that these claims were factually accurate. But they thought that these kinds of explanations, while true and important, did not provide a full representation of mindfulness.

Reflecting on the different political narratives through which mindfulness could be explained, Tom commented that, while mindfulness could not be reduced to resilience or well-being, the fact that different narratives could be used to frame it reflected its foundational nature:

> That's part of the versatility of narrative and the best articulation is a nuanced understanding that includes this array of character, grit, resilience, that kind of language, and recognises that we're dealing with complex concepts, because we're talking about a human potential that is multidimensional.

For Susan, narratives such as well-being and resilience did not capture the value of her personal practice.

> It's interesting, isn't it? Because I'm not sure I desperately connect with any of those words if I think about mindfulness and my own practice. Maybe 'well-being', but it's quite a vague term. 'Happiness' is an interesting one. Am I any happier through mindfulness? I'm not sure I'd use the word 'happy'. Happiness doesn't particularly resonate for what mindfulness does for me. 'Resilience' in some ways connects, but something around self-care and resilience rather than just that ability to bounce back. Perhaps for me 'resilience' in the past has been slightly brutal: 'Come on now, get back on the horse.' I think mindfulness in a way can enhance any of these different things. So, mindfulness might help happiness or resilience but I'm not sure it *is* resilience, or increased happiness.

Nonetheless, she thought that engaging skilfully with political narratives could point to a larger concern with 'living well':

> It isn't closing down. In some moments, resilience is what's needed, in other moments compassionate openness is what's needed. We need all these different qualities to actually navigate our lives and it's about flexibility and responsiveness and wider perspective taking, seeing what's most needed moment by moment. Yeah. And it's a nice way of framing it [. . .]. That's maybe moving it towards a bit of a narrative: what is it to live well.

Throughout the drafting process the need to explain mindfulness in terms of pragmatic outcomes and personal transformation remained present for volunteer advocates. Peter had a long-term meditation practice and he had been a key figure in the development of a popular meditation app. He and I took a walk along the canal in East London in the run-up to the general election of

2015. The towpath was busy with weekenders enjoying the spring weather and we stopped for a cup of tea on a narrow boat that had been refitted as a café. At this point in the drafting process, volunteers were struggling to find a language that would explain the value of mindfulness in political circles, to present mindfulness in such a way that what members thought of as its profoundly transformative potential could be understood by others. As he told me, 'What's starting to happen is we're finding words for why it is that much more important, but we're only just starting to do that. And so, you start by using the language that you *have* got like "well-being" or "resilience". And that's pretty visionary and big and cross-sector, but it's still kind of one set of language, one kind of frame'.

Useful Knowledge

The ethical value that mindfulness held for volunteers motivated their commitment to advocacy and maintained their belief in the broader political project of promoting mindfulness, but it occupied a subordinate position in the discursive hierarchy of the report itself. What made evidence for mindfulness 'useful' in the report was its ability to be communicated to and consumed by others (Strathern 2006, 75), and this was shaped by an idea of its 'users': the parliamentarians. The success of the document rested on its ability to assess mindfulness, provide accountability for political decisions that might be made as a result of it, and demonstrate value for money. As Susan told me in an interview after the report had been launched, 'What the politicians wanted was credibility. Something you could take to a minister and they would say, "This is really interesting."' The report needed to show that mindfulness was clearly supported by the evidence and costed for specific and targeted objectives.

For volunteer advocates, then, the presentation of mindfulness through econometric data and the evidence of randomised controlled trials did not feel disingenuous, but it did feel strategic. Peter, for example, understood the use of instrumental data as a way of communicating something of the value of mindfulness to people who had never practised it. He told me,

> Trying to describe mindfulness is a bit like trying to describe the taste of an orange. How do you do that? Okay, so it's hard to describe the taste of an orange, but you can point out the benefits of vitamin C. It protects you against colds, improves your skin, that sort of thing. That's sort of what we're doing: describing why it's socially important and the mechanisms it influences. But I think we can do better.

Peter understood the measurable effects of practising mindfulness, such as reduced cognitive reactivity, or emotional regulation, as secondary but important benefits of practice. But he focused on these measurable secondary benefits when presenting mindfulness as a policy object. Similarly, Teresa and others thought of mindful awareness as foundational for human flourishing and they did not think that the value of this could be completely accounted for by the evidence and targeted recommendations that they were compiling in the report. But, equally, they did not think of these metrics or the evidence that supported them as misleading or untrue. As Teresa said to me, 'that's the language you speak if you want to be part of the conversation'.

Over the course of drafting the report, volunteer advocates learned appropriate ways to represent mindfulness that were simultaneously moral and technical (see Harper 2000). They acted as knowledge brokers, bringing together information from think tanks, universities, research divisions and mental health institutes, in order to provide ideas and solutions with which policy makers could work. Drafting the report involved months of effort in reading research reports and collating their findings, discussing drafts and developing the text (see Harper 1998). The sheer amount of time and effort that went into getting the document 'right' is worth emphasising. I think of drafting the report as an ongoing social process, which was notable not only for the way in which novice advocates learned how to navigate the policy landscape, but also for the ways that it shaped mindfulness as a policy object. That is, through the writing process the 'parameters of the thinkable' (Green 2011, 42) were shaped. Explanatory practices were not just representational; they contributed to an iterative process which made it possible for mindfulness advocacy to develop, contributing to and shaping policy discussion in turn. In the service of explanation, evidence was marshalled and managed in order to establish 'what is the case' (ontological), to demonstrate 'how we know this is the case' (epistemological), and to develop a persuasive argument for 'what we think should be done' (normative). In the process, mindfulness *became* a policy object.

The final report made specific recommendations, supported by evidence, for how mindfulness could be introduced across UK services and institutions. In each policy area, the recommendations addressed identified policy objectives and were couched in emerging political narratives. Divided into four sections, the report presented a dizzying array of research. It provided pages of references detailing the nature and extent of problems identified in each area of the inquiry, and econometric data on the anticipated cost of these problems to the state. What had begun as a broad inquiry into mindfulness and mental health in the UK had now become an eighty-page comprehensive summary of much of the academic research on mindfulness at the time. The collation of this research had taken months to achieve and had orchestrated the efforts of a highly professionalised group of people. Mindfulness was presented as an evidence-based civil society recommendation with clear policy potential as a preventative healthcare intervention. It was framed as a possible solution to costed social problems, based on academic research which suggests that it 'works': statistical, social scientific and psychological research was marshalled to support the claim that mindfulness is an appropriate and positive intervention.

In addition to this, the report was prefaced with a two-page foreword by Jon Kabat-Zinn, the originator of MBSR (Mindfulness-Based Stress Reduction), and each of the key sections contained two to four pages of case studies of people who had benefited from mindfulness. The volunteers thought that both the foreword and the case studies were essential for the success of the document. Kabat-Zinn wrote that mindfulness 'has the potential to add value and new degrees of freedom to living life fully and wisely' (MAPPG 2015a, 9). Volunteers saw this representation of mindfulness as a 'way of being' that was cultivated 'wisely and effectively through practice' as a vital complement to the evidence-supported recommendations that made up the bulk of the report. In addition to the efficacy of mindfulness as a targeted intervention it was also, and importantly, represented as 'a way of being in wise and purposeful relationship with one's experience, both inwardly and outwardly' (ibid.). The case studies of people with health issues, a schoolgirl, a teacher, workers, a policeman, an ex-offender and a prisoner drew portraits of people who had learnt to 're-connect to life' and find time to 'simply be', in some cases in very challenging circumstances. Tom told me that, for him, it was these case studies that really communicated the value of mindfulness: sharing personal stories of the lived impact of mindfulness practice hit home powerfully. 'My hunch', he said, 'is that nobody really is inspired for a lifetime of mindfulness practice by randomised controlled trials and "resilience"; that it's as much a poetic enterprise as a scientific enterprise.'

In the animal protection charity studied by Adam Reed (2017b), personal ethical positions were articulated in political lobbying through the combination of scientific and moral techniques. Although photographic images and video footage of creatures caught in snares did not count as 'proper evidence' in political lobbying, campaigners presented both quantified evidence and visual representations of suffering animals in order to spark sympathy in politicians. Similarly, Deborah thought that the case studies in the report were important because they were *more* persuasive than the scientific evidence. As she said to me,

> What persuades who? Personal testimony. Because we're human beings, our hearts are engaged first and then our heads, and we always think we're persuaded by evidence but actually we seek the evidence once the case has caught us. But once we're persuaded, we need the evidence in order to go off and persuade others. But that gives us the confidence person to person to make it connect.

One effect of the creation of this document had been to shape a representation of mindfulness as an effective and evidence-based contribution to policy discussion not only about mental health, but also about well-being and resilience. Mindfulness was presented as a way of 'supporting wellbeing and resilience across the population as a prevention strategy to keep people well' (MAPPG 2015a, 19). This presentation of mindfulness as a preventative health measure was complemented by multiple research findings on the positive effects of mindfulness on cognitive and emotional processes, and a correlation was inferred between these processes and living a well-adjusted and happy life.

Conclusion: The Ethics and Economics of *Mindful Nation*

To conclude, I return to Lambek's distinction between ethical and economic value. As mindfulness is incorporated into political discussion, does it take on external values, rather than goods that were previously internal to it? Does a practice that was previously integrated into a total way of life come to be valued for the ends that it effects? One possible response might be that mindfulness is instrumentalised in the process of advocacy and comes to be valued for its goal-oriented efficacy. An alternative response might be that the presentation of mindfulness in utilitarian terms is disingenuous, and that its *real* value is as an ethical practice. I hope to have shown that neither interpretation is sufficient to account for the motivation for, and ongoing process of, political advocacy. My interest in this chapter has been to examine ethnographically the ways in which ethical and economic values (in Lambek's terms) intersect, and the efforts taken at different moments to maintain or reduce the distance between them. That is, rather than assuming that advocacy reduces the meaning of ethical value to a relative economic or utility value, I have asked, 'What is the ongoing relationship between ethical and economic value in the social process of advocacy?' The oil and water of ethical and economic values may be characteristic of contemporary political practice in the UK more broadly, and the incommensurability between the two may itself be productive. In the context of political advocacy, capacity and utility values are mutually reinforcing: if it were not for the evidence that it 'works', mindfulness would not be being discussed as a policy intervention; if the only value mindfulness had were extrinsic to it, advocates would not have sufficient moral conviction to campaign for it.

In accounting for the efforts that volunteer advocates made to draft the *Mindful Nation* report, I have sought to move away from a linear representation of political decision-making. Rather, political advocacy is revealed to be an ongoing and iterative social process. As Peter told me recently, 'political policies are like sausages: you wouldn't want to see how they get made'. Participation in mindfulness advocacy for non-state enthusiasts was motivated by personal moral conviction, and through marshalling multiple sources of evidence in the report, volunteers sought to contribute to cultural change. Volunteer advocates' efforts to explain the value of mindfulness in political conversations were intended as a political intervention. They did not just describe things in the world, but sought to explain to parliamentarians why these mattered and what should be done about them, and this explanation was achieved through the *management* of different kinds of evidence, drawing relationships between them and embedding them in broader political narratives. Volunteers learned to explain the value of mindfulness as a policy object through the collation of quantitative research, econometric data and the reproduction of what they understood to be prominent and salient discourses of the state. This led to what Kirsch has referred to (2008, 237) as a 'mimetic incorporation of bureaucratization', as volunteer advocates responded to the perceived nature of policy development and political conversation. I argue that engagement with governmental techniques that is motivated by personal ethics and located in broad normative agendas is informed by, coexists with and leads to multiple forms of rationality and ethics (see also Born 2002). The report may be thought of as a 'living document' (Green 2011)—a way of maintaining a place in an evolving conversation about policy, of navigating ongoing disputes and future possibilities. As such, it is alive with the social processes that produced it, and it continues to have a 'performative' quality even though the discursive form that it takes masks this 'politics of interaction' (see ibid.; Riles 2006).

By the end of my fieldwork in 2016, the inquiry process and the report had had relatively little impact on the policy landscape.[5] Nonetheless, the volunteers felt that their work had been a success: mindfulness had been put on the table and had become a staple in conversations about mental health in the UK. The massive public interest in mindfulness generated around the APPG and the *Mindful Nation* report were informed by and reflected in its uptake in the British press and in parliament. Volunteers saw advocating for mindfulness as part of a wider project of societal transformation, which was to be achieved by working with, rather than against, dominant political forms. Peter told me after the launch, 'This is our starter for ten, and then we begin the messy business of ongoing relationship-building and policy development over a number of years.' It is hard to know what the long-term effects of the *Mindful Nation* report will be in political terms, but at the time of the launch, Britain seemed to be on its way to becoming a mindful nation. Ironically (given the labour that went into collating the evidence), this had less to do with the development of specific policy 'asks' and more to do with a normalisation of debate about mental health and mindfulness that had occurred as a result of the process. At the end of the day, the promotion of the instrumentalised goals and targeted recommendations of the report had, in fact, led to a broad discussion about mental health and mindful awareness as constituent aspects of living well; an outcome that was in alignment with the ethical aspirations that had inspired the process of advocacy in the first place.

Keep Calm and Carry On?

I BEGAN CHAPTER 1 of this book with the launch of the *Mindful Nation* report at the end of 2015. The event marked the culmination of the APPG inquiry process, but it was also the most intense moment of a fast-paced and voracious media cycle centred on mindfulness. Throughout the period of my fieldwork, international media outlets published content about mindfulness at an unprecedented rate, fuelling intense public interest in meditation and mental health. The *Huffington Post* had labelled 2014 'the year of mindfulness' in a feature-length editorial (Gregoire 2014). In one of the most representative articles of the time, *Time* ran a cover story announcing the 'mindful revolution' (Pickert 2014). Mindfulness was presented as a way to 'find peace in a stressed-out, digitally dependent culture', a logical response to the contemporary malaise of 'distraction'. By giving oneself fully to what one is doing, '[o]ne can work mindfully, parent mindfully and learn mindfully. One can exercise and even eat mindfully. The banking giant Chase now advises customers on how to spend mindfully' (ibid.).

By the end of 2014, media interest in mindfulness was engaging with and outpacing the research. That mindfulness can reduce anxiety and depression was picked up on by the *Huffington Post* (Gregoire 2015); the *New York Times* emphasised that it improves quality of sleep (O'Connor 2015), and the *Harvard Gazette* highlighted that it can create measurable brain changes (McGreevey 2011). Media articles drew on research that suggested that mindfulness might help people pay attention (University of Miami 2014), make better decisions (Association for Psychological Science 2014) or maintain perspective (Teper and Inzlicht 2014). Readers of *Hello!* were told (*Hello!* 2014), 'If you're suffering from the winter blues or are feeling stressed and anxious, the solution could be all in the mind. To lift your mood with no side effects try meditation, not medication.' Citing the rising statistics on depression and the rise in antidepressant use in the UK, the article went on, 'You do not have to sit cross-legged on the floor, in robes, chanting a foreign language, instead, meditation involves taking time out to simply be—20 minutes a day is ideal.' A booming industry of popular books on the benefits of mindfulness and how to achieve them kept pace with this proliferation of column inches. As the buckling shelves in the well-being and self-help sections of bookshops attested, mindfulness was big business. The second edition of *Mindfulness for Dummies* was published in 2014 (Alidina 2014) and the ironic *Ladybird Book of Mindfulness* came out in 2015, which joked (Hazeley and Morris 2015, 6), 'There are now courses for cardio mindfulness, cockney mindfulness, honey-roast mindfulness and mindlessness. In mindlessness, you have to beat up your inner total stranger.'

If 2014 was the year of mindfulness, 2015 was, according to one *New York Times* article, the year of 'the mindfulness backlash' (North 2014). Media interest remained unremitting, but critiques from polar-opposite directions replaced the earlier tone of celebration. Mindfulness was criticised simultaneously for being too weak *and* too intensive. As a mental health intervention, it was described as 'papering over the cracks', a way of avoiding depression rather than resolving it, a quick cure-all or 'a sticking plaster that doesn't stick' (Hoggart 2015); a 'snack-sized approach [that] won't sort people out' (Barnett 2015; see also Nolan 2015). At the same time, others worried that the price of mindfulness might be 'madness' (Moody 2015), and that it could trigger 'twitching, trembling, panic, disorientation, hallucinations, terror, depression, mania and psychotic breakdown' (Wikholm and Farias 2015; see also Crawford 2015; Wilkholm 2015a). Other critics argued that mindfulness was both too Buddhist *and* not Buddhist enough. Mindfulness had either 'nosed its way into a secular audience' (Heffernan 2015), leading *Sky News* to ask, 'Should Buddhism be available on the NHS?' (Wikholm 2015b), or it was 'a form of Buddhism lite' (McDonagh 2015a; Heffernan 2015), and would 'do as much as a McDonald's Happy Meal to sate a person's gnawing hunger for a richer life' (Barnett 2015). The politics of mindfulness were criticised in similarly contradictory terms. It was both a left-wing conspiracy for systemic change, serving a naively transformative agenda (Michaelson 2014; Wikholm and Farias 2015), and a right-wing tool of neoliberal control, a selfish and 'mostly about me' (McDonagh 2014) way for 'one-percenters [. . .] to get even richer' (Michaelson 2014).

The people with whom I worked felt the effects of this mindfulness media cycle. Narratives in the media were filtering down into mindfulness therapists' classes and they were increasingly finding that they had to answer questions about mindfulness being either too Buddhist or not Buddhist enough, being either self-serving or a form of social control, being in the service of political agendas that were either left-wing and progressive or right-wing and capitalist, or being downright dangerous. By the first meeting of the parliamentary advocates in June 2014, the sheer scale of press interest in mindfulness was already evidently overwhelming for participants. Volunteer advocates were frequently asked for quotes from journalists on the benefits of mindfulness, a request about which many felt uneasy. They were deeply concerned that mindfulness was being presented as a cure-all, often with little understanding of what it is and what it entails. At the first meeting of the group, Sarah, the clinical research lead at a UK university, described media interest as a 'tsunami' and said that it was 'our responsibility to remain committedly unimpressed by media representations of mindfulness and its effects'. This was met by 'Hear, hear' around the room. Later, as we were saying our goodbyes, I asked her what she meant, and she told me that she saw no way to have a sensible conversation about mindfulness amid the chorus of media praise. 'Really,' she said, 'it's unsustainable; they're selling mindfulness as a panacea and it's not. There's got to be a backlash and I can only hope that it comes sooner rather than later. We need to be having a more balanced conversation.'

Sarah's wish for more critical engagement to temper the hyperbole was soon met, but rather than leading to the measured and productive conversation that she had hoped for, mindfulness became a media whipping boy. Throughout my fieldwork, this media over-hype and backlash proliferated. Mindfulness advocates were being contacted regularly for comment on the criticisms by the press. Throughout the backlash, mindfulness experts were asked to provide quotes and comments to feed the media interest. In each case they remained steadfastly unwavering in their message. In the *Financial Times*, Mark Williams was quoted as saying, 'There is a real danger of people being lured into thinking this is a cure for everything. [. . .] If people over-promise either to themselves or others, then they'll be over-disappointed' (Macaro and Baggini 2015). In the *Guardian*, Florian Ruths, a consultant psychologist at the South London and Maudsley NHS Foundational Trust, rejected the idea of mindfulness as 'fluffy or alternative', stating that it is an effective mental health treatment based on solid science (Berminham 2015). He also noted that it wasn't for everyone, particularly people who are acutely drug- and alcohol-dependent, recently bereaved, or in an acute episode of depression, but that side effects are rare.

This polarity between advocates and critics was reflected further in academic analyses. Supporters maintained that mindfulness prevents depressive relapse and reduces anxiety, that it increases empathic response, emotional regulation, higher cognitive functioning and attentional control, and that it is an important contributor to resilience, well-being and societal 'flourishing'. Critics of mindfulness argued that it is a form of neoliberal subjectification; that a previously ethically embedded practice had been reduced to a self-governance technique enslaved to neo-utilitarian values. They argued that mindfulness psychologises and individualises suffering, thereby leading to quietism by precluding the possibility of recognising misery as an effect of inequality, social injustice or political disenfranchisement (see further below).

A meeting of the advocates was called at the end of February 2016 to discuss the ways in which mindfulness was developing as a public object, and whether any response was required. The wave of negative press that mindfulness had received was troubling everyone. Where Sarah had once hoped for a more robust debate resulting from a media backlash, she now saw a discrepancy between the ways that mindfulness was being portrayed in the media and how people were engaging with mindfulness itself: 'If I look around, I see lots of grass-roots stuff that's countercultural; they're social enterprises, community projects, different ways of living as humans [. . .]. That's so different to what the media are saying.' It was agreed that the momentum and currency of the past two years had led to unprecedented interest in mindfulness, but that this was now leading to it being negatively caricatured. Mindfulness could be similarly critiqued from what were directly opposed positions (too Buddhist/not Buddhist enough, left-wing/right-wing, intensive/superficial) only because common representations of it relied on over-simplifying it, over-claiming it, or over-applying it. A former journalist reassured the meeting that, in her opinion, this was a media cycle and there was no way to respond to it:

This will just roll around and we have to ride it out. You can't respond to everything, and media culture now trades high in opinion based on very little knowledge. I don't think we've seen anything yet—people want a row. We need to keep a steady head and not get too involved in narratives. People's experience [of mindfulness] is what makes them advocates; we need to keep our feet on the ground.

The decision was taken at the meeting to retain equanimity in the face of media narratives, and it was agreed that it was impossible to fire-fight on all sides. As one of the clinical leads on mindfulness research told me in an interview afterwards, it was important to continue to present mindfulness in terms of both the universal and the specific vulnerability of being human. Mindfulness, she said, was a way 'to manage distress and work with it skilfully using the tool of the human mind', and press interest demanded a steady and level-headed response. This was echoed in the reflections of another volunteer advocate, as we mulled over the changing fortunes of mindfulness a few months later. Danny told me that he thought a decision was made 'to just keep sounding that note midst the cacophony of different voices, rather than feeling that you have to respond to all of them and it feels like it's a way to go crazy to feel you have to fight all the sides'. I asked him to expand on this, and he said that part of the challenge was that mindfulness could be framed in multiple ways:

> There will be critics on the right who see anything to do with meditation as just intrinsically left-wing hippy, just like there are people on the left who will see any self-governance project as an abdication of responsibility for changing social conditions. So it feels like there are pitfalls one has to avoid on both sides, but part of what's so interesting about it, and I guess I put it down to the very fundamental nature of metacognition and human activity, is that you can frame metacognition in multiple ways: you can frame it in terms of performance, you can frame it in terms of mental health, you can frame it in terms of relationship, you can frame it in terms of self-regulation; you know, it's the bedrock of human functioning: metacognition.

Danny's analysis of the public fortunes of mindfulness returns us to the centrality of metacognition as a support for mental health, but it also highlights the fact that the question of the proper relationship between psychological thinking and political practice is a highly contested domain. I have argued that psychological thinking underpins both practices of self-governance and governmental agendas, influencing how people make sense of their emotions, navigate everyday life, deliberate over public goods and promote social norms. This raises fascinating ethnographic questions about how psychological thinking informs the reimagining of psychological subjects, how techniques of governance are being reshaped and how the relationship between parliamentarians and citizen-subjects is reimagined through such techniques. In what follows, I develop a comparison between contemporary debate about mindfulness and an earlier psychologically informed political movement, the British second-wave feminist movement of the 1960s and 1970s, highlighting that in both cases, advocacy *and* critique form part of the complex dialogue by which psychological knowledge is incorporated into ethical and political frameworks. Examining advocacy for and critique of mindfulness through historical comparison highlights the contours of debate about psychological thinking in Britain, and enables us to reflect upon recent transformations in mental health, the valorisation of metacognition and the excitement about mindfulness that motivated the mindfulness practitioners who are at the heart of this book.

McMindfulness and Consciousness-Raising: Contesting Psychological Knowledge

The vanguard of the public critique of mindfulness was led by an early article in the *Huffington Post* (Purser and Loy 2013), in which mindfulness was caricatured by two academics as 'McMindfulness'. Purser and Loy argued that mindfulness is branded as 'Buddhist-inspired' because Buddhism has 'a certain cachet', but, shorn of its religious origins, commercialised mindfulness reinforces the greed, ill will and delusion institutionalised in the forces of modernity, amounting 'to a Faustian bargain':

> There is a dissociation between one's own personal transformation and the kind of social and organizational transformation that takes into account the causes and conditions of suffering in the broader environment. Such a colonization of mindfulness also has an instrumentalizing effect, reorienting the practice to the needs of the market, rather than to a critical reflection on the causes of our collective suffering.

'McMindfulness' is a pithy shorthand. It conveys the extinction of diversity in the face of unremitting capitalism, labelling people as addicted to patterns of consumption that keep them enslaved to the forces of modernity. It represents mindfulness as a homogeneous, dumbed-down, super-sized and nutritionally deficient but globally ubiquitous consumerist practice. This de-cultured, denatured, rebranded and repackaged mindfulness has lost its religious purpose and its cultural significance, rendering practitioners docile subjects of neoliberalism: pliable, sleepwalking free labour in a late capitalist era in which attention is harvested as if a crop (see also Reveley 2014). In short, mindfulness practices are dangerous (toxic, even), especially in corporate settings where they are employed to pacify manipulated and exploited workers, by shifting responsibility for stress onto individual employees, leading to quietism in oppressive working environments (see also Titmuss 2016). According to the critique, mindfulness is a panacea and a product that reproduces structures of social oppression by serving organisational agendas. The McMindfulness charge hits its mark on a regular basis. At the time of writing, Amazon is being lambasted on social media for installing 'AmaZen' booths in its factories— small telephone box-sized kiosks in which workers can 'focus on their mental wellbeing' by watching videos about mental health and mindfulness practices. These 'mindful practice rooms' have been sardonically christened 'cry closets' by workers who bear the brunt of poor working conditions, twelve-hour shifts, limited bathroom breaks and high injury rates (Kari 2021; Massie 2021).

Social-scientific studies of the use of psychological knowledge in governance have provided helpful critiques of the effects of inequality in human relations, the relationship between power and knowledge practices and the effects of categorisation and normalisation on the constitution and regulation of populations and people, and the McMindfulness critique reflects long-standing ideas: that therapeutic culture finds fertile ground in conditions of increasing consumerism (North 1972); that focusing on the psychological is a response to and a cause of the privatisation of life (Sennett 1977); that therapy is essentially narcissistic (Lasch 1980); and that psychological thinking is the basis of a new form of governance (Rose 1990). It is perhaps for this reason, along with the catchy name, that the McMindfulness critique has received significant press attention. It has been extended in subsequent academic publications (Purser 2015; Purser and Milillo 2015) and blogs (Purser and Ng 2015; Titmuss 2016), and was recently developed into a book aimed at popular audiences (Purser 2019). One recent edited volume, the somewhat misleadingly entitled *Handbook of Mindfulness* (Purser, Forbes and Burke 2016), sets out 'to expose how contemporary mindfulness programs are both compatible and complicit with neoliberal values' (ibid., x). Drawing on the early work of Foucault, the contributors argue that self-disciplinary regimes reproduce the workings of power and governmentality. In this analysis, mindfulness is a new form of bio-power in which 'the mind and the body become sites for self-disciplinary control, self-surveillance, and self-optimization' (ibid., xiv). Through this disciplinary apparatus, individuals not only 'voluntarily participate in their own governance, but also come to forget and forfeit bonds of solidarity and collectivity' (ibid., xiv; see also Caring-Lobel 2016; Ng 2016; Payne 2016; Walsh 2016). The editors conclude (2016, xvii) that '[t]he mindfulness revolution promises to bring relief and resolution to individuals debilitated by the demands of late capitalism, but without any political agenda, or any substantial challenge to the institutional structures which enable capitalism to inject its toxicity system-wide'. Mindfulness as an individual practice or as an organisational intervention is represented as a technique by which people adjust themselves to the injustices of their lives in order to better serve the interests of a capitalist social system.[1]

The parallels between the McMindfulness critique and earlier political engagement with psychological thinking are striking. In the former, we see a mobilisation of criticism in order to challenge prevailing social values and economic structures. The resulting critique of mindfulness acts as a vehicle for broader political mobilisation, in this case against neoliberal capitalism (broadly conceived) and critiquing mindfulness is framed as a heroic intervention, an opportunity to 'speak truth to power' (Purser, Forbes and Burke 2016). Likewise, British feminism of the 1960s and 1970s was also strongly influenced by the rejection of psychological intervention, identified as a form of social control. The popular work of psychiatrists such as R. D. Laing and Thomas Szasz, and the anti-psychiatry movement more broadly (see Laing 1969; Szasz 1961) had revealed the ways in which women were driven, literally, mad by the organisation of family life and had shown that psychiatry left 'disturbed' women in a state of dependency, reinforcing the femininity that was at the heart of their unhappiness (Thomson 2006). Furthermore, theories of psychological deprivation and child development were coming under fire for the extent to which they confused social and biological roles, thereby keeping mothers in the home. By the end of the 1960s, members of the women's movement were criticising psychology as a force for the oppression of women, challenging the association between psychology and the existing moral order to question the subordinate role of women in society (ibid., 279). The anti-psychiatric position acted as a rallying banner for the women's movement into the early 1970s, and labelling women as mentally ill was characterised as an act of political subjugation. As Thomson puts it, 'established theories and practices of psychology and psychiatry provided the women's movement with a powerful enemy to identify themselves against' (ibid., 280). And as Keane writes of the feminist movement in America (2016, 197),

> The identification of anger with the social category of women depends on a political analysis, but the way feminists care about it depends as well on an ethical vision of the good life. The politics is inseparable from the idea that a way of flourishing has been denied. It is on the basis of that sense that one's flourishing has been denied or thwarted that the feminist can link one distinct situation to another, treating both as instances of a single category: 'anger.'

Nevertheless, far from doing away with psychology altogether, both critiques reserve a central place for psychological thinking in politics. Psychological practice became central to the work of political liberation for the women's movement through the practice of 'consciousness-raising'. Through consciousness-raising sessions, women examined the details of their daily lives in order to make them explicit, such that they could be understood and subsequently addressed. Social transformation would result from bringing the details of personal experience into awareness, leading to commonality of purpose through the development of new group identities (oppressed women), whereby participants could understand themselves and relate to others. By focusing on the apparently trivial details of daily life, consciousness of oppression could be raised. As one reader wrote to the British feminist magazine *Spare Rib* in 1974, 'I have been led into believing I am crazy because I find it so difficult in a male orientated world. Then I read your magazine and I find I am right—life is hard, bloody hard.'[2] The psychological commonality of shared experience shifted responsibility from individual women to the social and political circumstances in which they found themselves. That is, psychological practices offered a means of creating a new politics and new values (Thomson 2006, 281).[3]

Similarly, the McMindfulness critique does not reject psychological knowledge or introspection altogether. Rather, its proponents call for a reconfiguration and a radicalisation of mindfulness as a political tool in the service of a socially interventionist agenda. By 'calling out' the axiological and political neutrality of mindfulness, the critique aims to enhance the common good by fostering 'civic and social mindfulness' (Purser, Forbes and Burke 2016, x). This interventionist project is premised on critique as the 'truth-telling' mechanism for societal improvement, without which we would remain in the maw of societal forces beyond ourselves. For example, Caring-Lobel argues (2016, 212) that '[i]t is high time we repoliticized stress and articulated our discontent, together'; and Ng calls (2016) for a 'critical mindfulness' as a disruptive technology of the self that might work against the dominant logics of the neoliberal capitalist order. At its base, then, the McMindfulness critique is normative: it is underpinned by a clear 'should'. It makes a case for why everyone should take up a *particular* psychologically informed political perspective, but it does not dismiss either mindfulness or the place of psychological thinking in social and political change. Mental health remains a universal concern, and introspection and metacognition are central to addressing it, but they are reconfigured as the means by which the politics of social change is enacted.

Practitioners should be engaging in political reflection through mindfulness practice, lest they succumb to the 'social amnesia that leads to mindful servants of neoliberalism' (Purser 2019, 23). Mindfulness, and by extension introspection, offers a possibility of an emancipatory politics through the incorporation of mindfulness into progressive social and political agendas, through which the structures of society might be challenged. As with the work of consciousness-raising, the call for a 'critical mindfulness' is based on a commitment to political critique through self-reflective work.

The comparison is helpful for drawing out the structure of contemporary media and academic debates about mindfulness. For some, mindfulness offers a hopeful and exciting moment of possibility. For others, it is a form of introspection that reaffirms the oppressive conditions of late capitalism. But a vision of psychological potential runs through *both* the promotion *and* the criticism of mindfulness. The potential of feminist consciousness-raising was similarly Janus-faced. Thomson (2006) highlights the inherent tensions in psychologically informed political action in the feminist movement: between being anti-psychiatric and yet embracing the psychological as crucial to personal transformation. In time, feminists distanced themselves from Laing and the anti-psychiatry position, which did little to address women's problems in their own right. And, as Thomson notes, women's accounts of struggle and depression that emerged through consciousness-raising practices challenged the anti-psychiatry movement's romanticisation of madness (2006, 281). But the tension between focus on the self and political action remained. For some, consciousness-raising offered the promise of mass mobilisation, a recognition of the social causes of suffering. For others, it was a means to personal self-realisation. The tension between these positions was difficult to reconcile. For feminists who prioritised social campaigning, consciousness-raising therapeutics could seem like a middle-class indulgence. For those focused on the internalisation of oppression, it was unclear what transformations in social conditions would be sufficient to address such deep-rooted psychological issues.

Debate about mindfulness similarly reflects different positions on the place of the psychological in political life. On the one hand, Purser argues (2019) that failing to address the societal causes of stress and collective suffering robs mindfulness of its revolutionary potential. On the other hand, the mindfulness advocate Jamie Bristow is representative of a counter-argument that while social conditions shape personal motivations, 'personal development is required for cultural development towards a more emotionally-intelligent, compassionate and just society' (Bristow 2019). It is possible that these debates reflect long-standing faultlines in psychological thinking in Britain more broadly: the notions either that personal development and introspection are vital if we are to tackle the complexity of contemporary societal challenges, or that they do nothing to address the social and economic inequalities that underpin them.[4] But they also point to the crossovers between professional, political and popular interest in psychological thinking. As we have seen in this book, the logics of preventative healthcare, the democratisation of mental health, the development of participatory governance, mindfulness advocacy and critique and media uptake of mindfulness all make dialogue across popular–political–professional divides particularly intense.

The Metacognitive Moment:
Self-Cultivation and the Promise of Psychology

The McMindfulness critique presents a picture very different from the one that has emerged through the ethnography of this book, in which people across society are excited by the potential of mindfulness to support them and others in living well, and engage with mindfulness as an ethical practice in their responses to the everyday challenges of mental health and daily life. Mindfulness is vast, it is engaged with by different people for different reasons and it is invested with multiple and often incommensurate values. As historian of religion Jeff Wilson writes of mindfulness in America (2014, 11), 'No matter where one stands, when looking into the mindfulness movement each observer is likely to find elements that strike him or her as crass, others that appear exploitative, things that are deeply moving, developments that seem genuinely positive, and phenomena that may be outright dangerous.' In this book, I have focused on mindfulness practitioners who are passionate about the potential of mindfulness as a support for living well. While significant numbers of people have heard of mindfulness, those who, like the people featured in this book, engage with it in a concerted way, either as an ethical practice, a therapy or a political object, will necessarily be in the minority. And, as we have seen in this chapter, contemporary enthusiasm about mindfulness in the press and in parliament is also met in those and other quarters by resistance, apathy and plain derision.

For the people featured in this book, however, excitement about supporting positively framed mental health, often lying well beyond the remit of professional psychology, informs their engagement with mindfulness. This excitement is reflected in the possibility and potentiality that has motivated British engagement with both psychology and Buddhism since the late nineteenth century (see chapter 1). As we have seen, the practitioners we have met in this book are excited about the psychological framing of mindfulness as they incorporate it into their daily activities, both as a therapeutic support (chapter 2) and as an ethical practice (chapter 3). We have also seen that mindfulness is modified through its relationship with broader sets of values and assumptions about human nature (chapter 4), that changing understandings about the good life influence the uptake of mindfulness across society and that this in turn informs changing modes of governance and governmental techniques in Britain (chapters 5 and 6). The promise mindfulness holds (not just for the individual, but also for society) transcends boundaries between the popular, professional and political, reflected in the 'common humanity' of the shift from the prevention of mental illness to the cultivation of mental health, the universalist framing of the insights of the psychological sciences and the logics of participatory governance. And it is reflected in changing aspirations for the good life: the prevention of depression, the reduction of harm or the minimisation of suffering, is expanded by optimism about living better, healthier, more fulfilling lives.

Mindfulness practitioners seek to relate to their minds in a particular way through the cultivation of a particular kind of metacognitive awareness. Through practice, the human capacity for reflection takes on a culturally specific form and value, one which combines intentional self-reflection with kindliness and compassion as a support for mental health. Anthropologists in the 'ethical turn' have theorised 'reflection' in different ways. Das (2012, 138) and Lambek (2015) recognise some kind of reflection as an important component in ordinary ethics. Keane (2010, 69) highlights the ways in which people step back from their lives in his distinction between first- and third-person perspectives (see Mattingly, 2014b, 26 for a comparative approach). As Keane writes (2016, 182), '[i]f self-distancing turns the flow of action into an *object* of thought, then this cognitive process of objectification, the third-person perspective it can produce, and the semiotic means that facilitate and sustain it are devices for ethical life'. Similarly, for Clarke (2016, 799), ethical reflection is 'utterly normal', and Robbins reminds us (2016) to focus on the reflective aspects of ethical life, rather than collapsing them into habit or 'culture' (see also Lambek 2000a). How we make sense of reflection, as a universal capacity informed by the particularities of specific contexts, and its relationship to practices of self-cultivation, is the focus of many of the debates in the anthropology of ethics (Heywood 2015; Keane 2016; Laidlaw 2014). As Heywood argues (2017, 44), such debates centre of the reconciliation between the universal and the particular: moral reasoning and reflection are universal capacities, and those capacities are contextually inflected. In the case of mindfulness, however, reflection is explicitly valorised, assuming normative status in its association with mental health: at root, the valorisation of metacognition is a call for transformations in people's awareness and self-awareness; taking a third-person perspective on experience (in Keane's terms) is unequivocally associated with flourishing and living well.

Anthropologists have highlighted that the ways in which people reflect upon themselves and seek to act are influenced by the particularities of specific contexts, and that there are at least some aspects of life that are self-directed and self-made (see Laidlaw 1995; Faubion 2001b; Robbins 2004). At the same time, they have highlighted the facts that action can be morally risky, that achievement can be precarious, and that humans are vulnerable to happenstance (Mattingly 2014b; Mittermaier 2011). They have shown that moral lives are complex, rarely homogeneous, and that people are often torn between diverse and sometimes conflicting values. The dialogic self-constitution of the subject in social relations reminds us that practices of self-cultivation occur in worlds that exceed that which might be shaped or influenced by the self. This does not negate, but rather emphasises the fact that people reflect on their circumstances and aspire to cultivate virtues in their responses to the vicissitudes of life. As Laidlaw argues (2014, 3), '[t]he claim on which the anthropology of ethics rests is not an evaluative claim that people are good: it is a descriptive claim that they are evaluative'. The question then becomes an empirical one: to enquire into the form and the extent of self-cultivation in specific lives without reducing it to a thin analysis of either atomistic individualism or social determinism (see also Cook 2023).

Such an approach offers a helpful perspective on the ways in which people reflect upon their experiences of mental health, and the effect that reflection has on the ongoing cultivation of mental health in the midst of life. In this book I have not represented people's experiences exclusively as effects of wider social forces, nor do I portray the people I worked with as managerial individuals, wholly responsible for the cultivation of their own psychological health. The people with whom I worked for over five years, from MBCT participants to parliamentarians, recognise their moral lives as being complex and plural, and what the 'good life' means for them is marked by competing ideas and values. They think that learning to relate to one's own mind with kindness is an important part of living well. For some, this is understood as preventing illness; for others it is understood as living more fully; for all, mental health is intentionally cultivated through practice in daily life. In itself, this book has been neither critical nor celebratory of mindfulness. Unlike some of my interlocutors, I do not imagine an end to the suffering of mental ill-health in the UK as a result of the spread and availability of mindfulness, though I do think that there are some people for whom it clearly offers a lifeline. But nor do I interpret the popularity of mindfulness as an effect and a perpetuation of social forces that colonise subjectivity. I hope to have shown that the relationship between models of mental health and the cultivation of a metacognitive relationship with one's own objectified mind informs the iterative relationship between subjectivity and political practice.

I have argued that paying attention to our minds has become a valued part of contemporary life, and that this has consequences for the ways in which we understand mental health and, therefore, what we ought to do about it. The development and widely perceived efficacy of mindfulness-based cognitive therapy for the prevention of depressive relapse made an important contribution to the contemporary popularity of mindfulness, but most people who practise mindfulness do not engage with it as a therapeutic intervention, and indeed have never received a mental health diagnosis. An increasing emphasis on preventative mental healthcare has expanded the meaning of 'mental health', swelling the populations for whom it is a relevant concern and transforming responses to address it. Combined, the logics of these developments have had a profound impact on the ways in which mental health is understood in the UK more broadly: mental health has become a transversal feature of life and one that can be actively supported through dedicated practices, such as mindfulness. And emphasis has shifted from illness to health: the prevention of illness is met and supported by the cultivation of positive mental health in order to 'live well'. Learning to relate to the mind in a healthy way has become a constitutive component of life, informed by prevalent social values and a sense of democratic and existential inclusivity. As we have seen, as mental health becomes a transversal concern, civil servants and politicians come to understand themselves as being as vulnerable to mental health issues as other British citizens, and the evidence from the psychological sciences is deliberated upon in political hearings as transversally relevant. Drawing on Hacking (1995a; 1995b; 2007), I have argued that transformations in the category of mental health have 'looping effects'. As increasing numbers of people come to understand their experiences through an expanded and reshaped understanding of mental health, the ways in which they describe these experiences change, as do the possible actions by which they might engage with, respond to or resist that experience. We have seen that the ways in which people represent mental health, the distinctions that they make and the solutions that those distinctions lead to have changed, and I have highlighted how the logics of preventative mental healthcare are incorporated into people's relationships with themselves, therapeutic interventions, structures of governance and political campaigns.

But I have also emphasised the cultural valorisation of metacognition—cultivating a kindly relationship with one's own objectified mind—as a support for mental health. This has ranged from effortful attention to the mind in therapeutic work and personal practice in everyday life to the working cultures and governmental techniques that inform an official political inquiry. It is a culturally novel phenomenon in the UK to think of the cultivation of attention and awareness, learning to develop a metacognitive relationship with one's own mind, as a central constituent of the good life. In this context, mindfulness practitioners invest the human capacity for reflection with culturally specific values. For the people at the heart of this book, mindfulness is both an instrumentalised, ameliorative intervention and an ethical practice; a pragmatic support for mental health and a 'way of being' that infuses everyday life. They think that mindfulness extends from formal practices into everyday life and that a healthy metacognitive relationship with oneself has a mutually constitutive relationship with virtuous dispositions of friendliness, patience and compassion. They also think that, properly validated, costed and communicated, mindfulness has the potential to help large numbers of people. In engagement with and promotion of mindfulness, this engagement with both ethical and economic values is maintained. The rationalism of scientifically grounded psychological services for the prevention and treatment of illness, and the Romanticism of the potential of self-work for living more fully, coalesce in the expanded category of mental health as a transversal issue and in the popularity of mindfulness as an evidence-based ethical practice.

NOTES

Introduction

1. For example, in his development of a continuum of mental health, Keyes defined 'languishing' as a condition of stagnation that does not constitute mental ill-health (2002a, 210; 2002b) and he defined 'flourishing' as referring to those 'individuals who have an enthusiasm for life and are actively and productively engaged with others and in social institutions'(2002a, 262).

2. Mindfulness has been shown to increase grey matter density (Hölzel, Carmody et al. 2011), improve positive affect (Moyer et al. 2011), and improve mental health outcomes (Hözel, Lazar et al. 2011). Studies suggest that mindfulness improves memory (Tang et al. 2007) and mental and physical stamina (McCracken and Yang 2008) and that meditation reduces the key indicators of chronic stress, including hypertension (Low, Stanton and Bower 2008), boosts the immune system (Davidson et al. 2003), and reduces the subjective experiences of chronic pain (Grant and Rainville 2009). Mindfulness has been shown to increase interpersonal empathy and compassionate responses to suffering (Condon et al., 2013). It has been related to a range of well-being constructs and is associated with enhanced self-awareness (Brown and Ryan 2003). Numerous studies suggest that meditators are happier than average (Ivanowski and Malhi 2007; Shapiro et al. 2008; Shapiro, Schwartz and Bonner 1998). And these findings are linked to a correlation between positive emotion, health and longevity (see Frederickson and Joiner 2002; Frederickson and Levenson 1998; Tugade and Frederickson 2004). And regular meditation has been shown to reduce anxiety, depression and irritability (Baer et al., 2006).

3. For example, Kuyken et al. had shown (2008) that MBCT was equivalent to maintenance antidepressants for the prevention of depressive relapse but was superior in terms of quality of life and residual depressive symptoms.

4. The universalising view underpinning this is that everyone would benefit from developing a decentred and healthy relationship with themselves by practising mindfulness, irrespective of their 'lower level' religious or social beliefs. The present moment takes on a primary or ontological status even though it has to be learned to be experienced. Mindful awareness of the present moment is framed as a human capacity, rather than as a propositional or cultural belief.

5. Scholarship in this area has been animated by an engagement with moral philosophy and a rethinking of Durkheim's profoundly influential sociology which established for British social anthropology an analytical focus on 'society': a structure which exists above and beyond, and encompasses, the people by whom it is constituted. Expressions of the collective will, such as customs, rules and laws, are compelling and desirable (see Durkheim 1953 [1906]). For Durkheim, morality imposes upon people the obligations which enable participation in the larger

social group; to be moral is to behave in accordance with social norms. Thus, what is good or right may be accounted for in the organisation of society, in the functional efficacy of its constituent parts and in moments of breach, in which social order breaks down (Laidlaw 2014, 28–29). This presents analysis with two challenges: firstly, it leaves no way to distinguish between 'moral' and 'social' behaviour, and secondly, it leaves no language to describe moral reasoning or ethical judgement. As Heywood puts it (2017, 45), '[i]f morality is simply what "society" tells you to do, and if whether you do it or not depends simply on whether "society" is or is not properly put together, then your capacity to think through the value, consequences, or virtue of doing it or otherwise is more or less redundant as far as the analyst is concerned.' (See too Parkin 1985, 4–5.)

Chapter 1

1. In charting a history of British engagement with Buddhist meditation, I seek to contribute to an evolving conversation about the genealogical roots of mindfulness. For example, excellent work has explored the history of relaxation as a forerunner to mindfulness (Nathoo 2019), the changing cultural value of equanimity (McKay 2019), projects of secularisation (Braun 2022), modernist Buddhism (McMahan 2008) and Buddhist sectarian influences on the development of mindfulness (Husgafvel 2018).

2. In his magisterial work, *The Making of Buddhist Modernism* (2008), David McMahan charts forms of Buddhism that emerged out of an engagement with modernity. Drawing on Taylor (1989), McMahan unpacks three discourses of modernity that have informed modernist renderings of the dharma: Western monotheism; rationalism and scientific naturalism; and Romantic expressivism. My focus on rationalism and Romanticism in the history of British engagement with Buddhism and psychology is deeply indebted to this work.

3. The Theosophical Society was strongly associated with Buddhist revivalism and presented a challenge to British evangelical missionary efforts established by the British colonial presence in Asia, most notably in the later work of London-born Annie Besant (1847–1933) in India.

4. Dreyfus and Thompson argue (2007, 94) that there is an affinity between James's 'introspective method' and Buddhist psychology. James took himself as the subject and object of investigations (James 1890), reflecting upon his everyday life experiences using 'retrospection' (remembering of a previous event). The method of 'normal psychology of introspection' (ibid., 194), in which the psychologist could be a commentator on their own experience, never took off as a psychological method. See Dryden and Still (2006) and Taylor (1991) on the multidirectional influence between James, humanistic psychology and Buddhism.

5. Pelmanism was a system of scientific mental training that promised to strengthen the mind. It was taught through correspondence courses and was popular in Britain in the first half of the twentieth century.

6. It is worth noting the striking contrast between this and interest in meditation in America at the time. In her history of the New Thought movement (2109), Hickey shows that religiously liberal concerns with the concentrated mind motivated the practice of meditation. New Thought leaders incorporated Buddhist and theosophical ideas into their explanations of mental healing and learned meditation from Buddhist and Hindu teachers (2019, 79–88). New Thought teachers and communities went on to promote meditation for physical, mental and spiritual healing, regularly recommending daily meditation (ibid., 63).

7. Concern over psychological subjectivity extended by 1939 into the arena of national and ideological warfare. Winning the Second World War would require defending national mental health as well as national borders, with the defence of British national character being itself a defence of democracy. Arguably, during this period psychological subjectivity became a political concern as never before. Yet this presented a paradox: national morale could not be defended through manipulative propaganda, as this was so closely associated with the power of dictators elsewhere in Europe and was therefore in ideological conflict with British liberal values. The response was an ideological commitment to rejection of overt psychological control and manipulation, and an emphasis on the appreciation of everyday life in the cultivation of psychological subjectivity (Thomson 1960, 227). But see Wu (2017, 37–50) for a discussion of highly successful British propaganda campaigns in advance of World War I.

8. For Gombrich and Obeyesekere, the widespread uptake of meditation by lay practitioners is the greatest single change in Theravāda Buddhist countries since the Second World War (1988, 237). Today this is a widely popular and influential movement, with vipassanā meditation being taught in monasteries and meditation centres throughout Thailand (Cook 2010a), Sri Lanka (Gombrich and Obeyesekere 1988), Burma (Jordt 2007) and Nepal (Gellner and LeVine 2005).

9. There is some disagreement about when this was first coined. Gethin (2011) traces it back to Rhys Davids (1881), while McMahan and Braun (2017) find it in a publication from 1877 (Rhys Davids 2000 [1877]).

10. Transcendentalism arose from English and German Romanticism in the late 1820s and 1830s in the United States. Core principles of transcendentalism include belief in the inherent goodness of people and nature, emphasising subjective intuition over objective empiricism, the power of the individual and personal freedom and an embracing of empirical science. Transcendentalism was strongly influenced by engagement with Asian religion and Versluis argues (2001, 3) that readings of the Bhagavad-Gita, the Vedas and the Upanishads were pivotal in the development of Transcendentalist thought. In 1844 the first English translation of the Lotus Sutra was published in The Dial, a publication of the New England Transcendentalists (Peabody 1844; see Lopez 2016), and a longing for intense spiritual experience through communion with nature influenced by Indian religion is reflected in Thoreau's writing in Walden (1854, 279): 'In the morning I bathe my intellect in the stupendous and cosmogonal philosophy of the Bhagavat Geeta [...]. I lay down the book and go to my well for water, and lo! there I meet the servant of the Brahmin, priest of Brahma, and Vishnu and Indra, who still sits in his temple on the Ganges reading the Vedas, or dwells at the root of a tree with his crust and water-jug. I meet his servant come to draw water for his master, and our buckets as it were grate together in the same well. The pure Walden water is mingled with the sacred water of the Ganges.'

11. In addition to the scientific study of meditation, meditation itself is also often conceived of as a proto-scientific technique, through which practitioners can observe their minds (see Cook 2017).

Chapter 2

1. Littlewood (1980) argued that normality and abnormality vary between cultures and societies (see Benedict 1934; Littlewood and Dein 1995) and that psychiatric classifications based on prototypes are singled out for culturally determined reasons (Littlewood and Lipsedge 1987). He examined the relationship between religion and symbolic classification, arguing that

'socially abnormal behaviour' may result from sets of culturally shared public symbols, which may vary between minority groups, and that rigid sets of Eurocentric classification cannot thus be relied on in an undifferentiated way. Littlewood's argument was extended by White and Marsella (1982), who argued that illness and abnormality are encompassed by cultural assumptions about the nature of persons and social behaviour.

2. Lutz, for example, in her work on the Ifaluk of Micronesia, challenged the tendency in Euro-American psychiatry to formulate depression as a dysfunction of the 'biopsychological' individual (1985, 69), rather than focusing on environment or interpersonal connectedness. Scheper-Hughes (1988) emphasised the ways in which 'nervous hunger' amongst poor Brazilians was informed by political meaning. Biehl (2005) understood the symptoms of a poor woman in Brazil, Katarina, as an ongoing and complicated resistance to an abusive marriage and family neglect. And Kirmayer (1991) interpreted the common Japanese psychiatric disorder *taijin kyofusho* as a pathological amplification of culture-specific concerns about impacting others' well-being through one's own improper conduct. (For excellent anthropological representations of culture and mental disorder, see Desjarlais 1994; Good 2012; Horwitz 2002.)

3. For anthropological analyses of chronicity in mental health, see Brodwin 2013; Davis 2012; Garcia 2008; Good et al. 2010; Luhrmann 2007; Manderson and Smith-Morris 2010.

4. For example, Nolen-Hoeksema and Morrow found (1991) that ruminative thinking patterns are associated with more prolonged depression.

5. Prior to the development of MBCT, Teasdale (1983) was attempting to understand the effects that mood has on thinking. Using short-lived mood inductions (by playing sad music or reading sad statements), he found that when induced into mild depressed moods, non-depressed people showed negative biases in memory (Teasdale, Taylor and Fogarty 1980).

6. In sequence: the right toes, the right foot, the right lower leg, the right knee joint, the right upper leg, the pelvic area, the lower back, the mid-back, the upper back and rib cage, the abdomen, chest, fingers, hands, lower arms, upper arms, shoulders, front neck, back neck, skull, head and face.

7. Sir David Attenborough is a veteran British broadcaster and naturalist. His combination of enthusiastic erudition, avuncular affability and breathy enunciation have made him a 'national treasure', with the ex-Monty Python comedian John Cleese even proposing him for benevolent dictator as a solution to democratic failure: https://twitter.com/johncleese/status /609034574774071296?lang=en (accessed 30 November 2022).

8. Dumit suggests (2002, 126–27) that genetic explanations acted as 'rhetorical barriers' to other candidates of causation such as society, environment or upbringing. These are relegated to secondary causes that may modify the genetic programmes that are the primary causes of illness: the environment 'triggers' the 'vulnerable' brain that is a product of genetic programming. This 'reinforces the sense that the real or proximate cause is the neurochemistry that is already predisposed toward the problem, waiting to be triggered'.

9. For an excellent overview of these debates, see O'Nell (1998).

10. For example, Kleinman's seminal work (see 1982; 1986) on somatisation and mental illness demonstrated that neurasthenia in China was informed by cultural and individual loss that resulted from the Cultural Revolution. On this basis, he argued that Chinese neurasthenia ought not be diagnosed as 'depression' despite parallels in symptomology, because this would mask insight into the cultural meaning of the experience. From this he drew his famous distinction

between 'disease' and 'illness' (disease being a biological malfunction, illness being the cultural and individual understanding of the disease).

11. For example, Young notes (1995) that Vietnam veterans were able to receive governmental compensation once they were recognised as suffering from PTSD, but, he argues, as a group they were left disenfranchised, because the PTSD discourse neutered the historical and political meaning of their experience.

12. Wells et al. (1996) measured disability in terms of 'days spent in bed'. They found that depressed patients took more 'duvet days' than patients with lung disease, diabetes or arthritis. Only patients with heart disease spent more time in bed.

13. Fifteen per cent of patients experiencing depressive symptoms severe enough to require hospitalisation are likely to die by suicide (Keller et al. 1992).

14. For moving accounts of depression, see also Lewis 2002; Solomon 2001; Wolpert 1999.

15. In O'Nell's work, Flathead depression extends beyond psychological distress into moral development, social relations, history and 'American Indian' identity as people seek to transform personal or collective demoralisation into positive moral character. Similarly, Throop (2010) highlighted the value of social suffering among the Yapese. In both cases, suffering, loss or loneliness are mediated through responsibility towards others, become central to social identity and are invested with powerful moral meanings.

16. On therapeutics as technologies of the self, see Martin 2010; McKinney and Greenfield 2010; Carr 2013.

17. For example, Horton (2017) shows that systems of psychiatric classification increasingly incorporate sociocultural issues into their classifications, reflecting the growing impact of cultural psychology and medical anthropology.

Chapter 3

1. While the everyday was an implicit focus in earlier social scientific work, on, for example, the atomisation of the metropolis for Simmel, the 'iron cage' or rationality for Weber or the monstrousness of modernity for Benjamin, from around the end of the twentieth century the category of the everyday gained increasing attention in the social sciences. Perhaps beginning with the influential publication in English of Michel de Certeau's *The Practice of Everyday Life* (1984 [1980]), the republication of English translations of Henri Lefebvre's works (1991 [1958]), and a return to the emphasis of the Frankfurt School upon the everyday as a focus for the study of modernity, subsequent scholarship has sought to problematise the meaning of everyday life itself.

2. As Clarke writes (2014, 418), 'just sticking a spike through your side will hardly do. It has to be done at the right time, in the right way, to an audience who, even if not captured by its proposition, at least understand the terms in which it is being proposed.'

3. The challenge of defining the 'ordinary' has been taken up in diverse ways by anthropologists in recent years. For example, in her work on ordinary ethics, Das (2012, 134) defines the 'ordinary' as against the 'transcendent'. Ethical work 'is done not by orienting oneself to transcendental, agreed-upon values but rather through the cultivation of sensibilities *within* the everyday' (emphasis in original); ethics are tacit as opposed to explicit, and found in the everyday. Similarly, in his programmatic essay on ordinary ethics (2010), Lambek defines ethics as

'ordinary' both in the sense of being 'basic to the human condition' and as immanent. For Lambek, 'the "ordinary" implies an ethics that is relatively tacit, grounded in agreement rather than rule, in practice rather than knowledge or belief, and happening without calling undue attention to itself' (2010, 2). Thus, ethical life is embedded in everyday practice as opposed to abstract rules or values (ibid., 2–3; see also Das 2010, 376–78; 2012). Here then, what makes ethics 'ordinary' is its immanence in interaction and its sheer everydayness: ethics is embedded in in the mundane, the quotidian. Others have challenged the immanence of 'ordinary' ethics, arguing that ethical life may require ongoing labour or may operate in different ethical modalities. For example, in a provocative critique of Lambek and Das, Lempert argues (2013) that assuming that ethics is necessarily tacitly present in the ground rules of interaction overlooks the performative contingency and labour that makes communication a precarious achievement. Taking a different tack, Keane argues that ethical life moves between different modalities, some of them tacit competences, others practices of objectification and deliberation, and thus 'ordinary' ethics are not always immanent. Stafford, meanwhile, follows Lambek in characterising ethical potential and demands as an 'ordinary' part of the human condition, observable in routine and everyday circumstances, often dealt with via tacit understanding (2013, 5), but he also views explicit ethical reflection as an 'ordinary' aspect of human life. He argues that, although ethics is sometimes located in the micro-processes of everyday life, it 'is also—routinely, ordinarily—the subject of explicit and conscious deliberation' (ibid.). Thus, for Stafford, ethics is 'ordinary' because it is sometimes tacit or immanent, and also because ethical reflection is entirely 'ordinary'. While the scholars cited here disagree about quality or quantity of 'immanence' in ordinary life, they share a commitment to the idea that ethics is found in the everyday. For example, Stafford adopts what he refers to as a 'small-is-beautiful approach' to the ordinary, focusing on what he refers to as the 'routine', the 'everyday' and the 'quotidian' in order to understand the ethical (2013, 6). For Keane and Lempert, ethical life may not be 'immanent', but it starts from 'sheer everydayness' and 'runs quietly through ordinary everyday activities' (Keane 2016, 17; see also Lempert 2013, 372). In his focus on the dynamics of 'everyday social interaction' (Keane 2016, 33) Keane writes (2010, 82), 'Both the tacit intimacy of habit and the vociferous distance of estrangement, the first person stance and the possibility of departing from it, are everyday conditions of life with other people.' On this point, Keane and Lempert are in agreement with Lambek and Das. Lambek considers 'everyday comportment and understanding' in his development of ordinary ethics. As he argues (2010, 3), 'the focus is less on special cases, unusual circumstances, new horizons, professional rationalizations, or contested forms of authorization than on everyday comportment and understanding'. For Das, even dramatic enactments of ethical value are grounded in the normative practices of everyday life (2012, 138). She considers the 'texture of everyday life', describing disappointment as the 'difficulty of reality in the 'ordinary realism' (2014, 488) of everyday struggle.

Chapter 4

1. Later published as Poulter et al. (2019).

2. IAPT is also the pathway through which NHS therapists train in Mindfulness-Based Cognitive Therapy (MBCT).

3. This genre of popular psychology is complemented by an equally bestselling strand of crossover scholarship which considers the ways in which forms of modern malaise result from social organisation; for example, as a result of increasing social isolation (Putnam 2000), keeping-up-with-the-Joneses (James 2007), or living in inequitable societies (Wilkinson and Pickett 2009).

4. Tracey Crouch was subsequently appointed minister for sport following the 2015 general election, a brief which was expanded to minister for civil society in June 2017, and she was appointed as the lead of a government-wide inquiry into loneliness in January 2018. She resigned as a minister in November 2018 over the timing of a £2 maximum stake on fixed-odds betting machines with the comment, 'Politicians come and go but principles stay with us forever' (see BBC News, 1 November 2018, https://www.bbc.co.uk/news/uk-politics-46057548 [accessed 30 November 2022]). She was also the first Conservative MP ever to take maternity leave.

5. The discourse of scientific Buddhism (McMahan 2008; McMahan and Braun 2017) has become increasingly sophisticated throughout the twentieth century, with numerous studies being produced on the relationship between Buddhism and science (see Dalai Lama 1999; 2004; Varela 1999; Wallace 2007).

6. The 'Irish backstop' was a proposed protocol to the 'Brexit' EU-withdrawal agreement. It aimed to prevent a hard border (with customs controls) between the Republic of Ireland and Northern Ireland after Brexit, but it never came into force.

Chapter 5

1. See 'Introduction' n. 1, above.

2. Large organisations such as the World Bank and the European Union have developed participatory governance practices, as have civil society organisations and charities such as Oxfam and Action Aid, and national government political parties. Principles of participatory governance are built into transdisciplinary research agendas and the collaborative incorporation of citizens in the work of scientific knowledge production (see Maasen and Lieven 2006). They are reflected in routine decision-making procedures in public administration (see Bora and Hausendorf 2010) and in new participatory fora and procedures such as public consultation exercises, consensus conferences, the incorporation of service users on advisory committees and the provision of public access to expert committees.

3. Critics of Evidence Based Medicine (EBM) have argued that a drive towards quantification and statistical analysis risks the loss of sensitivity to context and responsiveness to circumstance or individual patients (see Ecks 2008) with 'best evidence' increasingly defined by the data and analysis of RCTs (Williams and Garner 2002). By contrast, those in favour of EBM respond that preserving clinical autonomy perpetuates bias and personal preference in treatment protocols, thereby putting patients' health at risk. As Lambert points out (2005, 2640), arguments both for and against EBM often claim the moral high ground, in representing the greater good.

4. Or, as the 'Heads Up' campaign run by Heads Together with the FA (Football Association) (see https://www.headstogether.org.uk/heads-up/) told viewers nationwide in May 2019, 'Life often imitates football: we all experience setbacks from time to time, some big, some small, some

you see coming, others come out of the blue, and each setback puts our mental health to the test. So sometimes we need to take a moment to connect with the world around us.'

5. Here and elsewhere, the biggest challenge was finding financing for courses, with classes being initiated by prisons themselves and paid for out of prison budgets. Discussion about the implementation of mindfulness in prisons centred on the need to work sensitively with prison management and acknowledge the limits of budgets, time and space, and recognising the challenges of illiteracy and time management that presented barriers to participating in courses for some prisoners.

6. The preventative health turn emerged as part of a broader political-medical and cultural development focused on meeting the challenges of complicated health concerns through an emphasis on healthy quotidian behaviours. While some conditions, such as diabetes and hypertension, have a long history of successful pharmacological and lifestyle interventions, preventative strategies are increasingly considered appropriate for other forms of illness, such as late-onset Alzheimer's disease, and indeed ageing more broadly (see Lamb, Robbins-Ruszkowski and Corwin 2017; Leibing and Schicktanz 2021). For example, the emphasis now placed on 'ageing well' in North America and Europe reflects the impact of preventative healthcare across medical, public health, political and popular cultural narratives. Emphasising agency and choice, preventative approaches to old age encourage ageing well as a vital personal and moral project achieved through diet, exercise, productive activities, attitude, self-control and choice. As Lamb, Robbins-Ruszkowski and Corwin write (2017, 12), 'the successful aging movement is at once a morality tale, a medical tale, a governmental tale, and an existential tale, enacting cultural norms for persons as healthy, active, independent, and long-living subjects'. Similarly, dementia prevention reflects an increasing emphasis on 'lifestyle' as a support for positive health (see Foth 2021). Discourses of dementia prevention circulate in public discourse through a dialogue between communication channels such as popular science, clinical communication and internet fora (Schicktanz 2021).

Chapter 6

1. Tambiah (1990, 150) warns of similar effects of rationalisation when he writes that 'science invades the economy, the economy invades politics, and now politics is alleged to inform us on morality, choice and the values to live by. And there's the rub.'

2. Lambek argues that ethical values are posited in respect of absolute standards (the value of a life), while economic values fluctuate (economic value is negotiable). Furthermore, absolute values cannot be substituted for one another.

3. Viktor Frankl, an Austrian psychiatrist and Holocaust survivor, is commonly cited as writing, 'Between stimulus and response there is a space. In that space is our power to choose our response. In our response lies our growth and our freedom.' Despite the frequent attribution, the passage is not to be found in Frankl's writings. Frankl wrote a psychological memoir, *Man's Search for Meaning* (Frankl 2006 [1959]), in which he reflects on his experiences in Auschwitz, the purpose of life and courage in the face of difficulty. The quote was attributed to him by Stephen R. Covey in his bestselling self-help book *The Seven Habits of Highly Effective People* (1989), and it may be that the attribution entered common usage from there (see https://quoteinvestigator.com/2018/02/18/response/ [accessed 30 November 2022]).

4. The National Institute for Health and Care Excellence.

5. Within three years of the launch of the report, a series of actions had been taken that were indirectly linked to it. Two recommendations from the health chapter had been acted on: MBCT had become a mandated therapy through the IAPT (Improving Access to Psychological Therapies) programme, and Health Education England was funding MBCT therapist training. The Department for Education began funding a research trial on mindfulness and mental health interventions in schools. All of the report's recommendations in the criminal justice chapter were acted on, and the National Offender Management Service (now HMPPS [Her Majesty's Prison and Probation Service]) convened a steering group and conducted research on mindfulness among staff.

Conclusion

1. The McMindfulness analysis has received its fair share of criticism, with scholars and advocates arguing that there is no evidence that mindfulness practice leads to quietism (Lee 2019), that expecting mindfulness promotion to effect significant social change in pluralist societies is unrealistic (Schmidt 2016), that the critique misrepresents and exoticises the Buddhist antecedents of mindfulness (Anālayo 2020) and that it casts systemic change in an 'either/or' relationship with therapeutic approaches to distress (Bristow 2019).

2. Letter from Clair, 'Crazy Is as Crazy Is Done To', *Spare Rib*, 24 (1974), 3, cited by Thomson (2006, 280).

3. As Keane writes (2016, 196) of mid-century American feminist consciousness-raising, 'The anger becomes legitimate because the woman's current way of living turns out not to be the only one available. New possibilities, new ways of being a woman—what virtue ethics would call new kinds of human flourishing—have emerged. By making these possibilities explicit, these sessions made them available for people to recognize in other people and other circumstances and to respond with criticism, enthusiasm, hostility, support, or just plain confusion.'

4. It is possible that the existence of the McMindfulness critique is a sign of weakness, as much as of strength, of the neoliberal psychological state (see also Thomson 2006, 267), and that, given its promotion in popular media, the critique itself acts as a brake on the kinds of development that it bemoans. That is, in arguing that mindfulness acts as a means of social control, whether or not it is, figures such as Purser limit public receptivity to the psychological vision of those who champion mindfulness.

BIBLIOGRAPHY

Abraham, Charles and Susan Michie. 2008. 'A Taxonomy of Behaviour Change Techniques Used in Interventions'. *Health Psychology* 27: 379–87.

Adler, Nancy E., Thomas Boyce, Margaret A. Chesney, Sheldon Cohen, Susan Folkman, Robert L. Kahn and Leonard S. Syme. 1994. 'Socioeconomic Status and Health: The Challenge of the Gradient'. *American Psychologist* 49 (1): 15–24.

Albanese, Catherine. 2007. *A Republic of Mind and Spirit: A Cultural History of American Metaphysical Religion*. New Haven, CT: Yale University Press.

Alexandrova, Anna. 2017. *A Philosophy for the Science of Well-Being*. New York: Oxford University Press.

Alfano, Mark. 2013. *Character as Moral Fiction*. Cambridge: Cambridge University Press.

Alidina, Shamash. 2014. *Mindfulness for Dummies* (2nd edition). Chichester: Wiley.

Almond, Philip C. 1988. *The British Discovery of Buddhism*. Cambridge: Cambridge University Press.

Anālayo, Bhikku. 2020. 'The Myth of McMindfulness'. *Mindfulness* 11: 472–79.

Anderson, Amanda. 2018. *Psyche and Ethos: Moral Life after Psychology*. Oxford: Oxford University Press.

Arden, John B. 2010. *Rewire Your Brain: Think Your Way to a Better Life*. Hoboken, NJ: Wiley.

Arnold, Edwin. 2009 [1879]. *The Light of Asia: or The Great Renunciation, Being the Life and Teaching of Gautama, Prince of India and Founder of Buddhism*. New York: Cosimo Classics.

Ashdown, (Lord) P(addy) (chair). 2011. *Humanitarian Emergency Response Review*. Available at https://www.preventionweb.net/publication/humanitarian-emergency-response-review (accessed 30 November 2022).

Association for Psychological Science. 2014. 'Mindfulness Meditation May Improve Decision-Making, New Study Suggests'. *ScienceDaily*, 12 February, https://www.sciencedaily.com/releases/2014/02/140212112745.htm (accessed 30 November 2022).

Baer, Ruth A. 2003. 'Mindfulness Training as a Clinical Intervention: A Conceptual and Empirical Review'. *Clinical Psychology: Science and Practice* 10: 125–43.

Baer, Ruth A., Gregory T. Smith, Jaclyn Hopkins, Jennifer Kreitemeyer and Leslie Toney. 2006. 'Using Self-Report Assessment Methods to Explore Facets of Mindfulness'. *Assessment* 13: 27–45.

Bajaj, Badri and Neerja Pande. 2016. 'Mediating Role of Resilience in the Impact of Mindfulness on Life Satisfaction and Affect as Indices of Subjective Well-Being'. *Personality and Individual Differences* 93: 63–67.

Barnett, Emma. 2015. 'Mindfulness: The Saddest Trend of 2015'. *The Telegraph*, 8 January. Available at https://www.telegraph.co.uk/women/womens-life/11331034/Mindfulness-the-saddest-trend-of-2015.html (accessed 30 November 2022).

Barrios, Roberto E. 2016. 'Resilience: A Commentary from the Vantage Point of Anthropology'. *Annals of Anthropological Practice* 40 (1): 28–38.

Batchelor, Stephen. 1994. *The Awakening of the West: The Encounter of Buddhism and Western Culture*. London: Aquarian Press.

Baumann, Martin. 2002. 'Buddhism in Europe: Past, Present, Prospects'. In *Westward Dharma: Buddhism beyond Asia*, edited by Charles S. Prebish and Martin Baumann, 85–105. Berkeley, CA: University of California Press.

Beck, Ulrich. 1992. *Risk Society: Towards a New Modernity*. London: Sage.

Bender, Courtney. 2010. *The New Metaphysicals: Spirituality and the American Religious Imagination*. Chicago: University of Chicago Press.

Benedict, Ruth. 1934. 'Anthropology and the Abnormal'. *Journal of General Psychology* 10 (1): 59–82.

Berman, Marshall. 2009. *All That Is Solid Melts into Air: The Experience of Modernity*. New York: Verso.

Bermingham, Kate. 2015. 'Mindfulness: An Effective Mental Health Treatment but not a Panacea'. *The Guardian*, 14 May. Available at https://www.theguardian.com/healthcare-network/2015/may/14/mindfulness-mental-health-treatment-nhs (accessed 30 November 2022).

Biehl, João. 2005. *Vita: Life in a Zone of Social Abandonment*. Berkeley, CA: University of California Press.

Bishop, Scott R., Mark Lau, Shauna Shapiro, Linda Carlson, Nicole D. Anderson, James Carmody, Zindel V. Segal et al. 2004. 'Mindfulness: A Proposed Definition'. *Clinical Psychology: Science and Practice* 11: 230–41.

Blanchot, Maurice. 1993. *The Infinite Conversation*, translated by Susan Hanson. Minneapolis: University of Minnesota Press.

Bluck, Robert. 2008. *British Buddhism: Teachings, Practice and Development*. London: Routledge.

Bora, Alfons and Heiko Hausendorf (eds). 2010. *Democratic Transgressions of Law: Governing Technology through Public Participation*. Leiden: Brill.

Born, Georgina. 2002. 'Reflexivity and Ambivalence: Culture, Creativity and Government in the BBC'. *Cultural Values* 6: 65–90.

Borup, Jørn. 2008. 'Buddhism in Denmark'. *Journal of Global Buddhism* 9: 27–37.

Braun, Erik. 2013. *The Birth of Insight: Meditation, Modern Buddhism, and the Burmese Monk Ledi Sayadaw*. Chicago: University of Chicago Press.

Braun, Erik. 2017. 'Mindful but not Religious: Meditation and Enchantment in the Work of Jon Kabat-Zinn'. In *Meditation, Buddhism and Science*, edited by David L. McMahan and Erik Braun, 172–97. Oxford: Oxford University Press.

Braun, Erik. 2022. 'Seeing through Mindfulness Practices'. In *The Oxford Handbook of Buddhist Practice*, edited by Kevin Trainor and Paula Arai, 632–48. Oxford: Oxford University Press.

Bristow, Jamie. 2019. 'Time for New Thinking about Mindfulness and Social Change'. *Open Democracy*, 3 September, https://www.opendemocracy.net/en/transformation/time-new-thinking-about-mindfulness-and-social-change/ (accessed 30 November 2022).

Brodwin, Paul. 2013. *Everyday Ethics: Voices from the Front Line of Community Psychiatry.* Berkeley, CA: University of California Press.

Brown, Phil. 1995. 'Naming and Framing: The Social Construction of Diagnosis and Illness'. *Journal of Health and Social Behavior* 35: 34–52.

Brown, Wendy. 2003. 'Neo-liberalism and the End of Liberal Democracy'. *Theory and Event* 7 (1): 1–21.

Brown, Kirk. W. and Richard. M. Ryan. 2003. 'The Benefits of Being Present: Mindfulness and Its Role in Psychological Well-Being'. *Journal of Personality and Social Psychology* 84 (4): 822–48.

Cadge, Wendy. 2005. *Heartwood: The First Generation of Theravada Buddhism in America.* Chicago: University of Chicago Press.

Caduff, Carlo. 2010. 'Public Prophylaxis: Pandemic Influenza, Pharmaceutical Prevention and Participatory Governance'. *BioSocieties* 5 (2): 199–218.

Caring-Lobel, Alex. 2016. 'Corporate Mindfulness and the Pathologization of Workplace Stress'. In *Handbook of Mindfulness: Culture, Context, and Social Engagement,* edited by Ronald E. Purser, David Forbes and Adam Burke, 195–214. Basel: Springer.

Carlson, Linda E. 2012. 'Mindfulness-Based Interventions for Physical Conditions: A Narrative Review Evaluating Levels of Evidence'. *ISRN Psychiatry,* https://doi.org/10.5402/2012/651583.

Carr, E. Summerson. 2013. 'Signs of Sobriety: Rescripting American Addiction Counseling'. In *Addiction Trajectories,* edited by Eugene Raikhel and William Garriott, 160–87. Durham, NC: Duke University Press.

Cassaniti, Julia. 2016. *Living Buddhism: Mind, Self, and Emotion in a Thai Community.* Ithaca, NY: Cornell University Press.

Cassaniti, Julia 2018 *Remembering the Present: Mindfulness in Buddhist Asia.* Ithaca, NY: Cornell University Press.

Cassaniti, Julia and Tanya M. Luhrmann 2014 'The Cultural Kindling of Spiritual Experiences'. *Current Anthropology* 55 (S10): S333–43.

Cassaniti, Julia L. and Usha Menon 2017 'Introduction'. In *Universalism without Uniformity: Explorations in Mind and Culture,* edited by Julia Cassaniti and Usha Menon, 1–22. Chicago: University of Chicago Press.

Certeau, Michel de. 1984 [1980]. *The Practice of Everyday Life,* translated by Steven F. Rendall. Berkeley, CA: University of California Press.

Chandler, David. 2014. *Resilience: The Governance of Complexity.* London: Routledge.

Chase, Liana. 2019. 'Healing 'Heart-Minds': Disaster, Care and Global Mental Health in Nepal's Foothills'. Doctoral thesis, SOAS University of London.

Chiesa, Alberto and Alessandro Serretti. 2009. 'Mindfulness-Based Stress Reduction for Stress Management in Healthy People: A Review and Meta-analysis'. *The Journal of Alternative and Complementary Medicine* 15 (5): 593–600.

Clark, David Alexander 2002. *Visions of Development: A Study of Human Values.* Cheltenham: Edward Elgar.

Clarke, Morgan. 2014. 'Cough Sweets and Angels: The Ordinary Ethics of the Extraordinary in Sufi Practice in Lebanon'. *JRAI* 20 (3): 407–25.

Clarke, Morgan. 2016. 'Comment' [on Robbins 2016]. *JRAI* 22 (4): 797–99.

Coelho, H. F., P. H. Canter and E. Ernst. 2007 'Mindfulness-Based Cognitive Therapy: Evaluating Current Evidence and Informing Future Research'. *Journal of Consulting and Clinical Psychology* 75, 1000–1005.

Condon, Paul, Gaëlle Desbordes, Willa B. Miller and David DeSteno. 2013. 'Meditation Increases Compassionate Responses to Suffering'. *Psychological Science* 24 (10): 2125–27.

Cook, Joanna. 2010a. *Meditation in Modern Buddhism: Renunciation and Change in Thai Monastic Life*. Cambridge: Cambridge University Press.

Cook, Joanna. 2010b. 'Ascetic Practice and Participant Observation; or, The Gift of Doubt and Incompletion in Field Experience'. In *Emotions in the Field: Surviving and Writing-Up Fieldwork Experience*, edited by James Davies and Dimitrina Spencer, 239–65. Stanford, CA: Stanford University Press.

Cook, Joanna. 2015. 'Detachment and Engagement in Mindfulness-Based Cognitive Therapy'. In *Detachment: Essays on the Limits of Relational Thinking*, edited by Matei Candea, Joanna Cook, Catherine Trundle and Thomas Yarrow, 219–35. Manchester: Manchester University Press.

Cook, Joanna. 2016. 'Mindful in Westminster: The Politics of Meditation and the Limits of Neoliberal Critique'. *HAU: Journal of Ethnographic Theory* 6 (1): 69–91.

Cook, Joanna. 2017. '"Mind the Gap": Appearance and Reality in Mindfulness-Based Cognitive Therapy'. In *Meditation, Buddhism, and Science*, edited by David L. McMahan & Erik Braun, 114–32. Oxford: Oxford University Press.

Cook, Joanna. 2018. 'Paying Attention to Attention'. *Anthropology of This Century* 22. http://aotcpress.com/articles/paying-attention-attention/ (accessed 30 November 2022).

Cook, Joanna. 2020. 'Unsettling Care: Intersubjective Embodiment in MBCT'. *Anthropology and Humanism* 45 (2) (special issue: *Unsettled Care*, edited by Joanna Cook and Catherine Trundle): 184–93.

Cook, Joanna. 2023. 'Self-Cultivation'. In *The Cambridge Handbook of the Anthropology of Ethics and Morality*, edited by James Laidlaw. Cambridge: Cambridge University Press.

Cooper, David. 1967. *Psychiatry and Anti-psychiatry*. London: Tavistock Publications.

Covey, Stephen R. 1989. *The Seven Habits of Highly Effective People*. New York: Simon & Schuster.

Crawford, Harriet. 2015. 'The Dark Side of Meditation and Mindfulness: Treatment Can Trigger Mania, Depression and Psychosis'. *The Daily Mail*, 22 May. Available at https://www.dailymail.co.uk/health/article-3092572/The-dark-meditation-mindfulness-Treatment-trigger-mania-depression-psychosis-new-book-claims.html (accessed 30 November 2022).

Crisp, Roger and Brad Hooker (eds). 2000. *Well-Being and Morality: Essays in Honour of James Griffin*. Oxford: Oxford University Press.

Cruikshank, Barbara. 1996. 'Revolutions Within: Self-Government and Self-Esteem'. In *Foucault and Political Reason*, edited by Andrew Barry, Thomas Osborne and Nikolas Rose, 231–51. Chicago: University of Chicago Press.

Culadasa (John Yates), and Matthew Immergut. 2015. *The Mind Illuminated: A Complete Meditation Guide Integrating Buddhist Wisdom and Brain Science for Greater Mindfulness*. Pearce, AZ: Dharma Treasure Press.

Cummins, Robert A. 2005. 'Measuring Health and Subjective Wellbeing: Vale, Quality-Adjusted Life-Years'. In *Rethinking Wellbeing*, edited by Lenore Manderson and Richard Nile, 69–89. Perth, W.A.: API Network.

Cush, Denise. 1996. 'British Buddhism and the New Age'. *Journal of Contemporary Religion* 11 (2): 195–208.

Cushman, Philip. 1995. *Constructing the Self, Constructing America: A Cultural History of Psychotherapy*. Reading, MA: Addison-Wesley.

Dafoe, Terra and Lana Stermac. 2013. 'Mindfulness Meditation as an Adjunct Approach to Treatment within the Correctional System'. *Journal of Offender Rehabilitation* 52 (3): 198–216.

Dalai Lama, The 14th. 1999. *Consciousness at the Crossroads: Conversations with the Dalai Lama on Brain Science and Buddhism*, edited by Zara Houshmand, Robert B. Livingston and B. Alan Wallace. Ithaca, NY: Snow Lion.

Dalai Lama, The 14th. 2004. *New Physics and Cosmology: Dialogues with the Dalai Lama*, edited by Arthur Zajonc with Zara Houshmand. New York: Oxford University Press.

Danziger, Kurt. 1990. *Constructing the Subjects: Historical Origins of Psychological Research*. New York: Cambridge University Press.

Das, Veena. 2010. 'Engaging the Life of the Other: Love and Everyday Life'. In *Ordinary Ethics: Anthropology, Language, and Action*, edited by Michael Lambek, 376–99. New York: Fordham University Press.

Das, Veena. 2012. 'Ordinary Ethics'. In *A Companion to Moral Anthropology*, edited by Didier Fassin, 133–49. Malden, MA: Wiley-Blackwell.

Das, Veena. 2014. 'Ethics, the Householder's Dilemma, and the Difficulty of Reality'. *HAU: Journal of Ethnographic Theory* 4 (1): 487–95.

Dasgupta, Partha. 2001. *Human Well-Being and the Natural Environment*. Oxford: Oxford University Press.

Davidson, Richard J., Jon Kabat-Zinn, Jessica Schumacher, Melissa Rosenkranz, Daniel Muller, Saki. F. Santorelli, Ferris Urbanowski, Anne Harrington, Katherine Bonus and John F. Sheridan. 2003. 'Alterations in Brain and Immune Function Produced by Mindfulness Meditation'. *Psychosomatic Medicine* 65: 564–70.

Davies, Huw T. O., Sandra M. Nutley and Peter C. Smith (eds). 2000. *What Works? Evidence-Based Policy and Practice in Public Services*. Bristol: Polity Press.

Davis, Elizabeth Anne. 2012. *Bad Souls: Madness and Responsibility in Modern Greece*. Durham, NC: Duke University Press.

Department of Health. 2005. *The National Service Framework for Mental Health: Five Years On*. London: Department of Health.

Department of Health. 2008. *High Quality Care for All: NHS Next Stage Review Final Report*. Available at https://webarchive.nationalarchives.gov.uk/ukgwa/20130105053023/http://www.dh.gov.uk/en/Publicationsandstatistics/Publications/PublicationsPolicyAndGuidance/DH_085825 (accessed 30 November 2022).

Department of Health. 2009. *NHS 2010–2015: From Good to Great: Preventative, People-Centred, Productive*. Available at https://webarchive.nationalarchives.gov.uk/ukgwa/20130105084309/http://www.dh.gov.uk/en/Publicationsandstatistics/Publications/PublicationsPolicyAndGuidance/DH_109876 (accessed 30 November 2022).

Desjarlais, Robert. 1994. 'Struggling Along: The Possibilities for Experience among the Home-less Mentally Ill'. *American Anthropologist* 96: 886–901.

Doris, John M. 2002. *Lack of Character: Personality and Moral Behavior*. Cambridge: Cambridge University Press.

Dreyfus, George and Evan Thompson. 2007. 'Asian Perspectives: Indian Theories of Mind'. In *The Cambridge Handbook of Consciousness* edited by Phillip D. Zelazo, Morris Moscovitch and Evan Thompson, 89–114. Cambridge: Cambridge University Press.

Dryden, Windy and Arthur Still. 2006. 'Historical Aspects of Mindfulness and Self-Acceptance in Psychotherapy'. *Journal of Rational Emotive and Cognitive Behaviour Therapy* 24 (1): 3–28.

du Gay, Paul. 2005. 'The Values of Bureaucracy: An Introduction'. In *The Values of Bureaucracy*, edited by Paul du Gay, 1–13. Oxford: Oxford University Press.

Dumit, Joseph. 2002. 'Drugs for Life'. *Molecular Interventions* 2 (3): 124–27.

Durkheim, Émile. 1953.[1906]. 'The Determination of Moral Facts'. In Émile Durkheim, *Sociology and Philosophy*, translated by D. F. Pocock, 35–60. New York: The Free Press.

Ecks, Stefan. 2005. 'Pharmaceutical Citizenship: Antidepressant Marketing and the Promise of Demarginalization in India'. *Anthropology and Medicine* 12 (3): 239–54.

Ecks, Stefan. 2008. 'Three Propositions for an Evidence-Based Medical Anthropology'. *JRAI* 14 (S1) (special issue: *The Objects of Evidence: Anthropological Approaches to the Production of Knowledge*, edited by Matthew Engelke): 77–92.

Elliott, Carl. 2018. 'Does your Patient Have a Beetle in his Box? Language-Games and the Spread of Psychopathology'. In *The Grammar of Politics: Wittgenstein and Political Philosophy*, edited by Cressida J. Heyes, 186–201. Ithaca, NY: Cornell University Press.

Epstein, Steven. 1996. *Impure Science: AIDS, Activism, and the Politics of Knowledge*. Berkeley, CA: University of California Press.

Eyal, Gil, Brendan Hart, Emine Onculer, Neta Oren and Natasha Rossi. 2010. *The Autism Matrix: The Social Origins of the Autism Epidemic*. Cambridge: Polity Press.

Farquhar, Judith and Qicheng Zhang. 2012. *Ten Thousand Things: Nurturing life in Contemporary Beijing*. New York: Zone Books.

Faubion, James. 2001a. 'Toward an Anthropology of Ethics: Foucault and the Pedagogies of Autopoesis'. *Representations* 74: 83–104.

Faubion, James. 2001b. *The Shadow and Lights of Waco: Millennialism Today*. Princeton, NJ: Princeton University Press.

Federman, Asaf. 2015. 'Buddhist Meditation in Britain: 1853 to 1945'. *Religion* 45 (4): 553–72.

Feldman, Christina and Willem Kuyken. 2011. 'Compassion in the Landscape of Suffering'. *Contemporary Buddhism* 12 (1): 143–55.

Foth, Thomas. 2021. 'Governing through Prevention: Lifestyle and the Health Field Concept'. In *Preventing Dementia? Critical Perspectives on a New Paradigm of Preparing for Old Age* edited by Annette Leibing and Silke Schicktanz, 214–41. New York: Berghahn Books.

Foucault, Michel. 1984. 'What is Enlightenment?' In *The Foucault Reader*, edited by Paul Rabinow, 32–50. New York: Pantheon Books.

Foucault, Michel. 1994. 'Nietzsche, Genealogy, History'. In *The Essential Works of Foucault 1954–1984*, vol. 2: *Aesthetics*, edited by James D. Faubion, 369–91. New York: The New Press.

Foucault, Michel. 1997. 'What Is Enlightenment?' In *The Essential Works of Michel Foucault 1954–1984*, vol. 1: *Ethics: Subjectivity and Truth*, edited by Paul Rabinow, 303–19. New York: The New Press.

Frankl, Viktor. 2006 [1959]. *Man's Search for Meaning*. Boston, MA: Beacon Press.

Franklin, Sarah. 2003. 'Ethical Biocapital: New Strategies of Cell Culture'. In *Remaking Life and Death: Toward an Anthropology of the Biosciences*, edited by Sarah Franklin and Margaret Lock, 97–127. Santa Fe, NM: School of American Research Press.

Frederickson, Barbara. L. and Thomas Joiner. 2002. 'Positive Emotions Trigger Upward Spirals toward Emotional Well-Being'. *Psychological Science* 13: 172–75.

Fredrickson, Barbara. L. and Robert W. Levenson. 1998. 'Positive Emotions Speed Recovery from Cardiovascular Sequelae of Negative Emotions'. *Cognition and Emotion* 12: 191–220.

Gajaweera, Nalika. 2016. 'What's So Wrong with Mindfulness?' *Tricycle: The Buddhist Review*, Winter (vol. 27 no. 2). Available at https://tricycle.org/magazine/whats-wrong-mindfulness/ (accessed 30 November 2022).

Garcia, Angela. 2008. 'The Elegiac Addict: History, Chronicity, and the Melancholic Subject'. *Cultural Anthropology* 23 (4): 718–46.

Geertz, Clifford. 1975. 'Common Sense as a Cultural System'. *The Antioch Review* 33 (1): 5–26.

Gellner, David N. and Sarah LeVine. 2005. *Rebuilding Buddhism: The Theravada Movement in Twentieth-Century Nepal*. Cambridge, MA: Harvard University Press.

Gellner, Ernest. 1960. *Words and Things*. London: Routledge.

Gethin, Rupert. 2011. 'On Some Definitions of Mindfulness'. *Contemporary Buddhism* 12 (1): 263–79.

Gilpin, Richard. 2008. 'The Uses of Theravada Buddhist Practices and Perspectives in Mindfulness-Based Cognitive Therapy'. *Contemporary Buddhism* 9 (2): 227–51.

Goleman, Daniel and Richard Davidson. 2018. *The Science of Meditation: How to Change Your Brain, Mind and Body*. London: Penguin.

Gombrich, Richard and Gananath Obeyesekere. 1988. *Buddhism Transformed: Religious Change in Sri Lanka*. Princeton, NJ: Princeton University Press.

Good, Byron. 2012. 'Theorizing the 'Subject' of Medical and Psychiatric Anthropology'. *JRAI* 18 (3): 515–35.

Good, Byron J. and Mary-Jo DelVecchio Good. 1982. 'Toward a Meaning-Centred Analysis of Popular Illness Categories: 'Fright Illness' and 'Heart Distress' in Iran'. In *Cultural Conceptions of Mental Health and Therapy*, edited by Anthony J. Marsella and Geoffrey M. White, 141–66. Dordrecht: Reidel.

Good, Byron J., Mary-Jo DelVecchio Good and Robert Moradi. 1985. 'The Interpretation of Iranian Depressive Illness and Dysphoric Affect'. In *Culture and Depression: Studies in the Anthropology and Cross-cultural Psychiatry of Affect and Disorder*, edited by Arthur Kleinman and Byron J. Good, 369–428. Berkeley, CA: University of California Press.

Good, Byron J., Carla Raymondalexis Marchira, Nida Ul Hasanat, Muhana Sofiati Utami and Subandi. 2010. 'Is "Chronicity" Inevitable for Psychotic Illness? Studying Heterogeneity in the Course of Schizophrenia in Yogyakarta, Indonesia'. In *Chronic Conditions, Fluid States: Globalization and the Anthropology of Illness*, edited by Lenore Manderson and Carolyn Smith-Morris, 54–74. Ithaca, NY: Rutgers University Press.

Gordon, James E. 1978. *Structures: Or Why Things Don't Fall Down*. Harmondsworth: Penguin.

Gottweis, Herbert. 2008. 'Participation and the New Governance of Life'. *BioSocialities* 3 (3): 265–86.

Grant, Joshua. A. and Pierre Rainville. 2009. 'Pain Sensitivity and Analgesic Effects of Mindful States in Zen Meditators: A Cross-sectional Study'. *Psychosomatic Medicine* 71 (1): 106–14.

Green, Maia. 2011. 'Calculating Compassion: Accounting for Some Categorical Practices in International Development'. In *Adventures in Aidland: The anthropology of professionals in international development*, edited by David Mosse, 33–56. Oxford: Berghahn.

Gregoire, Carolyn. 2014. 'Why 2014 Will Be the Year of Mindful Living'. *Huffpost* (UK edition), 2 January, updated 17 January 2017, https://www.huffingtonpost.co.uk/entry/will-2014-be-the-year-of_n_4523975 (accessed 30 November 2022).

Gregoire, Carolyn. 2015. 'How Mindfulness is Revolutionising Mental Health Care'. *Huffpost* (UK edition), 23 January, updated 23 February, https://www.huffingtonpost.co.uk/entry/neuroscience-mindfulness_n_6531544?ri18n=true (accessed 30 November 2022).

Griffin, James. 1986. *Well-Being: Its Meaning, Measurement and Moral Importance*. Oxford: Oxford University Press.

Grinker, R. R. 2007. *Unstrange Minds: Remapping the World of Autism*. New York: Basic Books.

Hacking, Ian. 1995a. 'The Looping Effects of Human Kinds'. In *Causal Cognition: A Multidisciplinary Approach*, edited by Dan Sperber, David Premack and Ann J. Premack, 351–94. Oxford: Clarendon Press.

Hacking, Ian. 1995b. *Rewriting the Soul: Multiple Personality and the Sciences of Memory*. Princeton, NJ: Princeton University Press.

Hacking, Ian. 1999. *The Social Construction of What?* Cambridge, MA: Harvard University Press.

Hacking, Ian. 2007. 'Kinds of People: Moving Targets.' *Proceedings of the British Academy* 151: 285–318.

Haidt, Jonathan. 2001. 'The Emotional Dog and Its Rational Tail: A Social Intuitionist Approach to Moral Judgment'. *Psychological Review* 108 (4): 814–34.

Haidt, Jonathan. 2006. *The Happiness Hypothesis: Putting Ancient Wisdom and Philosophy to the Test of Modern Science*. London: Heinemann.

Hallisey, Charles. 2014. 'Roads Taken and Not Taken in the Study of Theravāda Buddhism'. In *Defining Buddhism(s): A Reader*, edited by Karen Derris and Natalie Gummer, 92–117. New York: Routledge.

Hanson, Rick. 2009. *Buddha's Brain: The Practical Neuroscience of Happiness, Love, and Wisdom*. Oakland, CA: New Harbinger Publications.

Harper, Richard. 1998. *Inside the IMF: An Ethnography of Documents, Technology and Organisational Action*. San Diego, CA: Academic Press.

Harper, Richard. 2000. 'The Social Organization of the IMF's Mission Work: An Examination of International Auditing'. In *Audit Cultures: Anthropological Studies in Accountability, Ethics and the Academy*, edited by Marilyn Strathern, 23–53. London: Athlone.

Hazeley, Jason and Joel Morris. 2015. *The Ladybird Book of Mindfulness*. London: Penguin.

Healy, David. 1997. *The Antidepressant Era*. Cambridge, MA: Harvard University Press.

Hedegaard, Holly, Sally C. Curtin and Margaret Warner. 2020. 'Increase in Suicide Mortality in the United States, 1999–2018'. *NCHS Data Brief 362*, https://www.cdc.gov/nchs/data /databriefs/db362-h.pdf (accessed 30 November 2022).

Hedegaard, Marianne. 2020. 'The Mindful Gardener and the Good Employee'. In *Buddhism and Business: Merit, Material Wealth, and Morality in the Global Market Economy*, edited by Trine Brox and Elizabeth Williams-Oerberg, 93–110. Honolulu: University of Hawai'i Press.

Heffernan, Virginia. 2015. 'The Muddied Meaning of "Mindfulness"'. *The New York Times Magazine*, 14 April. Available at https://www.nytimes.com/2015/04/19/magazine/the-muddied -meaning-of-mindfulness.html (accessed 30 November 2022).

Helderman, Ira. 2019. *Prescribing the Dharma: Psychotherapists, Buddhist Traditions, and Defining Religion*. Chapel Hill: University of North Carolina Press.

Hello!. 2014. 'Think Happy'. *Hello! Magazine*, February (anon.).

Heywood, Paolo. 2015. 'Freedom in the Code: The Anthropology of (Double) Morality'. *Anthropological Theory* 15: 200–217.

Heywood, Paolo. 2017. 'Moral Psychology: An Anthropological Perspective'. In *Moral Psychology: A Multidisciplinary Guide*, edited by B. Voyer and T. Tarantola, 43–58. New York: Springer.

Heywood, Paolo. 2022. 'Ordinary Exemplars: Cultivating the Everyday in the Birthplace of Fascism'. *Comparative Studies in Society and History* 64 (1): 91–121.

Heywood, Paolo and Matei Candea (eds). 2023. *Beyond Description: Anthropologies of Explanation*. Ithaca, NY: Cornell University Press.

Hickey, Wakoh Shannon. 2010. 'Two Buddhisms, Three Buddhisms, and Racism'. *Journal of Global Buddhism* 11: 1–25.

Hickey, Wakoh Shannon, 2019. *Mind Cure: How Meditation Became Medicine*. Oxford: Oxford University Press.

Highmore, Ben. 2002. *Everyday Life and Cultural Theory: An Introduction*. London: Routledge.

Himelstein, Sam, Arthur Hastings, Shauna Shapiro, and Myrtle Heery. 2012. 'Mindfulness Training for Self-Regulation and Stress with Incarcerated Youth: A Pilot Study'. *Probation Journal* 59: 151–65.

Hirschbein, Laura. 2014. *American Melancholy: Constructions of Depression in the Twentieth Century*. New Brunswick, NJ: Rutgers University Press.

Hirschkind, Charles. 2001. 'The Ethics of Listening: Cassette-Sermon Audition in Contemporary Cairo'. *American Ethnologist* 28 (3): 623–49.

Hirschkind, Charles. 2006. *The Ethical Soundscape: Cassette Sermons and Islamic Counterpublics*. New York: Columbia University Press.

Hoesterey, James Bourk. 2016. *Rebranding Islam: Piety, Prosperity, and a Self-Help Guru*. Stanford, CA: Stanford University Press.

Hoggett, Paul. 2005. 'A Service to the Public: The Containment of Ethical and Moral Conflict by Public Bureaucracies'. In *The Values of Bureaucracy*, edited by Paul du Gay, 165–90. Oxford: Oxford University Press.

Hoggart, Philip. 2015. 'Be Mindful of Mindfulness: Drug-Free Doesn't Mean Side-Effect Free'. *The Guardian*, 21 May. Available at https://www.theguardian.com/science/brain-flapping /2015/may/21/mindfulness-drug-free-side-effects (accessed 30 November 2022).

Holling, Crawford S. 1973. 'Resilience and Stability of Ecological Systems'. *Annual Review of Ecology and Systematics* 4: 1–23.

Hollon, Steven D. and Philip C. Kendall. 1980. 'Cognitive Self-Statements in Depression: Development of an Automatic Thoughts Questionnaire'. *Cognitive Therapy and Research* 4: 383–95.

Hölzel, Britta K., James Carmody, Mark Vangel, Christina Congleton, Sita M.Yerramsetti, Tim. Gard and Sara W. Lazar. 2011. 'Mindfulness Practice Leads to Increases in Regional Brain Gray Matter Density'. *Psychiatry Research: Neuroimaging* 191: 36–43.

Hölzel, Britta K., Sara. W. Lazar, Tim Gard, Zev Schuman-Olivier, David R. Vago and Ulrich Ott. 2011. 'How Does Mindfulness Meditation Work? Proposing Mechanisms of Action from a Conceptual and Neural Perspective'. *Perspectives on Psychological Science* 6: 537–59.

Horton, Randall. 2017. 'Cultural Psychology and the Globalization of Western Psychiatric Practices'. In *Universalism without Uniformity: Explorations in Mind and Culture*, edited by Julia Cassaniti and Usha Menon, 241–59. Chicago: University of Chicago Press.

Horwitz, Allan. 2002. *Creating Mental Illness*. Chicago: University of Chicago Press.

Horwitz, Allan V. and Jerome C. Wakefield. 2007. *The Loss of Sadness: How Psychiatry Transformed Normal Sorrow into Depressive Disorder*. Oxford: Oxford University Press.

Humphreys, Christmas. 2012 [1974]. *Exploring Buddhism* (reprint edition). London: Routledge.

Huppert, Felicia A. 2005. 'Positive Mental Health in Individuals and Populations'. In *The Science of Well-Being*, edited by Felicia. A. Huppert, Nick Baylis and Barry Keverne, 307–40. Oxford: Oxford University Press.

Huppert, Felicia A. 2009. 'A New Approach to Reducing Disorder and Improving Well-Being'. *Perspectives on Psychological Science* 4 (1): 108–11.

Husgafvel, Ville. 2018. 'The "Universal Dharma Foundation" of Mindfulness-Based Stress Reduction: Non-Duality and Mahāyāna Buddhist Influences in the Work of Jon Kabat-Zinn'. *Contemporary Buddhism* 19 (2): 275–326.

Hyland, Terry. 2016. '*Mindful Nation UK*—Report by the Mindfulness All-Party Parliamentary Group (MAPPG)'. *Journal of Vocational Education and Training* 68 (1): 133–36.

Ingleby, David 1980. *Critical Psychiatry: The Politics of Mental Health*. New York: Pantheon.

Ivanowski, Belinda and Gin S. Malhi. 2007. 'The Psychological and Neurophysiological Concomitants of Mindfulness Forms of Meditation'. *Acta Neuropsychiatrica* 19: 76–91.

Jackson, Mark. 2013. *The Age of Stress: Science and the Search for Stability*. Oxford: Oxford University Press.

Jacob, Marie-Andrée and Annelise Riles. 2007. 'The New Bureaucracies of Virtue: Introduction'. *Political and Legal Anthropology Review* 30 (2): 181–91.

James, Oliver. 2007. *Affluenza: How to be Successful and Stay Sane*. London: Vermillion.

James, William. 1890. *The Principles of Psychology*, 2 vols. London: MacMillan.

James, William. 2020 [1902]. *Varieties of Religious Experience*. New York: Editorium.

Jasanoff, Sheila (ed.). 1994. *Learning from Disaster: Risk Management after Bhopal*. Philadelphia: University of Pennsylvania Press.

Jasanoff, Sheila. 2003. 'Technologies of Humility: Citizen Participation in Governing Science'. *Minerva* 41: 223–44.

Jeffries, Stuart. 2008. 'Will This Man Make You Happy?'. *The Guardian*, 24 June. Available at https://www.theguardian.com/lifeandstyle/2008/jun/24/healthandwellbeing.schools (accessed 30 November 2022).

Jordt, Ingrid. 2007. *Burma's Mass Lay Meditation Movement: Buddhism and the Cultural Construction of Power*. Athens, OH: Ohio University Press.

Josefsson, Torbjörn, Pernilla Larsman, Anders G. Broberg and Lars-Gunnar Lundh. 2011. 'Self-Reported Mindfulness Mediates the Relation between Meditation Experience and Psychological Well-Being'. *Mindfulness* 2: 49–58.

Jung, Carl. 1961. *Memories, Dreams, Reflections*, edited by Aniela Jaffé, translated by Richard and Clara Winston. New York: Random House.

Kabat-Zinn, Jon. 1982. 'An Outpatient Program in Behavioral Medicine for Chronic Pain Patients Based on the Practice of Mindfulness Meditation: Theoretical Considerations and Preliminary Results'. *General Hospital Psychiatry* 4 (1): 33–47.

Kabat-Zinn, Jon. 1994. *Wherever You Go There You Are: Mindfulness Meditation in Everyday Life*. New York: Hyperion.

Kabat-Zinn, Jon. 2005. *Coming to Our Senses: Healing Ourselves and the World through Mindfulness*. New York: Hyperion.

Kabat-Zinn, Jon. 2011. 'Some Reflections on the Origins of MBSR, Skillful Means, and the Trouble with Maps'. *Contemporary Buddhism: An Interdisciplinary Journal* 12 (1): 281–306.

Kabat-Zinn, Jon. 2013 [1990]. *Full Catastrophe Living: Using the Wisdom of Your Body and Mind to Face Stress, Pain, and Illness*. New York: Bantam Books.

Kahneman, Daniel. 2011 *Thinking, Fast and Slow*. London: Penguin Books.

Kari, Paul. 2021. 'Amazon's Mental Health Kiosk Mocked on Social Media as a "Despair Closet"', *The Guardian*, 28 May. Available at https://www.theguardian.com/technology/2021/may/27/amazons-mental-health-kiosk-mocked-on-social-media-as-a-despair-closet (accessed 30 November 2022).

Karp, David A. 1996. *Speaking of Sadness: Depression, Disconnection, and the Meanings of Illness*. New York: Oxford University Press.

Keane, Webb. 2010. 'Minds, Surfaces, and Reasons in the Anthropology of Ethics'. In *Ordinary Ethics: Anthropology, Language, and Action*, edited by Michael Lambek, 64–83. New York: Fordham University Press.

Keane, Webb. 2016. *Ethical Life*. Princeton, NJ: Princeton University Press.

Keller, Martin B., Philip W. Lavori, Collins E. Lewis, and Gerald L. Klerman. 1983. 'Predictors of Relapse in Major Depressive Disorder'. *Journal of the American Medical Association* 250: 3299–304.

Keller, Martin B., Philip W. Lavori, Timothy I. Mueller, William Coryell, Robert M. A. Hirschfeld and Tracie Shea. 1992. 'Time to Recovery, Chronicity and Levels of Psychopathology in Major Depression'. *Archives of General Psychiatry* 49: 809–16.

Kelly, Tobias. 2008. The Attractions of Accountancy: Living an Ordinary Life during the Second Palestinian *Intifada*. *Ethnography* 9 (3): 351–76.

Kessler, Ronald C., Patricia Berglund, Olga Demler, Robert Jin, Kathleen R. Merikangas and Ellen E. Walters. 2005 'Lifetime Prevalence and Age-of-Onset Distributions of DSM-IV Disorders in the National Comorbidity Survey Replication'. *Archives of General Psychiatry* 62: 593–602.

Keyes, Charles F. 1985. 'The Interpretive Basis of Depression'. In *Culture and Depression: Studies in the Anthropology and Cross-cultural Psychiatry of Affect and Disorder*, edited by Arthur Kleinman and Byron J. Good. Berkeley, CA: University of California Press: 153–74.

Keyes, Corey L. M. 2002a. 'Promoting a Life Worth Living: Human Development from the Vantage Points of Mental Illness and Mental Health. In *Promoting Positive Child, Adolescent and Family Development: A Handbook of Program and Policy Innovations*, edited by Richard M. Lerner, Francine Jacobs and Donald Wertlieb, vol. 4: *Adding Value to Youth and Family Development: The Engaged University and Professional and Academic Outreach*, 257–74. Thousand Oaks, CA: Sage.

Keyes, Corey L. M. 2002b. 'The Mental Health Continuum: From Languishing to Flourishing in Life'. *Journal of Health and Social Behavior* 43: 207–22.

Kim-Cohen, Julia, Avshalom Caspi, , Terrie E. Moffitt, Hona Lee Harrington, Barry J. Milne and Richie Poulton. 2003. 'Prior Juvenile Diagnoses in Adults with Mental Disorder: Developmental Follow-Back of a Prospective Longitudinal Cohort'. *Archives of General Psychiatry* 60: 709–17.

Kirmayer, Laurence. 1991. 'The Place of Culture in Psychiatric Nosology: *Taijin kyofusho* and DSM-III-R'. *The Journal of Nervous and Mental Disease* 179 (1): 19–28.

Kirmayer, Laurence J. 2006. 'Culture and Psychotherapy in a Creolizing World'. *Transcultural Psychiatry* 43 (2): 163–68.

Kirmayer, Laurence J. 2015a. 'Mindfulness in Cultural Context'. *Transcultural Psychiatry* 52 (4): 447–69.

Kirmayer, Laurence J. 2015b. 'Re-visioning Psychiatry: Toward an Ecology of Mind in Health and Illness'. In *Re-visioning Psychiatry: Cultural Phenomenology, Critical Neuroscience, and Global Mental Health*, edited by Laurence J. Kirmayer, Robert Lemelson and Constance A. Cummings. Cambridge: Cambridge University Press.

Kirsch, Thomas G. 2008 *Spirits and Letters: Reading, Writing and Charisma in African Christianity*. New York: Berghan Books.

Kitanaka, Junko. 2011. *Depression in Japan: Psychiatric Cures for a Society in Distress*. Princeton, NJ: Princeton University Press.

Kleinman, Arthur. 1982. 'Neurasthenia and Depression: A Study of Somatization and Culture in China'. *Culture, Medicine and Psychiatry* 6: 117–90.

Kleinman, Arthur. 1986. *Social Origins of Distress and Disease: Depression, Neurasthenia, and Pain in Modern China*. New Haven, CT: Yale University Press.

Kleinman, Arthur. 1988. *Rethinking Psychiatry: From Cultural Category to Personal Experience*. New York: The Free Press.

Kleinman, Arthur. 2004. 'Culture and Depression'. *The New England Journal of Medicine* 351 (10): 951–53.

Kleinman, Arthur and Byron Good. 1985. *Culture and Depression: Studies in the Anthropology and Cross-cultural Psychiatry of Affect and Disorder*. Berkeley, CA: University of California Press.

Kleinman, Arthur and Joan Kleinman. 1985. 'Somatization: The Interconnections in Chinese Society among Culture, Depressive Experiences, and the Meanings of Pain'. In *Culture and Depression: Studies in the Anthropology and Cross-cultural Psychiatry of Affect and Disorder*, edited by Arthur Kleinman and Byron Good, 429–90. Berkeley, CA: University of California Press.

Kleinman, Arthur, Yunxiang Yan, Jing Jun, Sing Lee, Everett Zhang, Pan Tianshu, Wu Fei and Guo Jinhua. 2011. *Deep China: The Moral Life of the Person; What Anthropology and Psychiatry Tell Us about China Today*. Berkeley, CA: University of California Press.

Kornfield, Jack. 1977. *Living Buddhist Masters*. Kandy: Buddhist Publication Society.

Kousoulis, Antonis. 2019. *Prevention and Mental Health: Understanding the Evidence so We Can Address the Greatest Health Challenge of Our Times*. Mental Health Foundation. Available at https://www.mentalhealth.org.uk/sites/default/files/2022-06/MHF-Prevention-report -2019.pdf (accessed 30 November 2022).

Kuan, Teresa. 2015. *Love's Uncertainty: The Politics and Ethics of Child Rearing in Contemporary China*. Oakland: University of California Press.

Kuyken, Willem, Sarah Byford, Rod S. Taylor, Ed Watkins, Emily Holden, Kat White, Barbara Barrett, Richard Byng, Alison Evans, Eugene Mullan, and John D. Teasdale. 2008. 'Mindfulness-Based Cognitive Therapy to Prevent Relapse in Recurrent Depression'. *Journal of Consulting and Clinical Psychology* 76: 966–78.

Labour Party. 2015. *Labour Party Manifesto 2015: Britain Can Be Better*. Available at https://manifesto .deryn.co.uk/labour-manifesto-2015-britain-can-be-better/ (accessed 30 November 2022).

Laidlaw, James. 1995. *Riches and Renunciation: Religion, Economy, and Society among the Jains*. Oxford: Clarendon Press.

Laidlaw, James. 2002. 'For an Anthropology of Ethics and Freedom'. *JRAI* 8 (2): 311–32.

Laidlaw, James. 2014. *The Subject of Virtue: An Anthropology of Ethics and Freedom*. Cambridge: Cambridge University Press.

Laing, Ronald D. 1969. *The Divided Self: An Existential Study in Sanity and Madness*. London: Tavistock Publications.

Lamb, Sarah, Jessica Robbins-Ruszkowski and Anna I. Corwin. 2017. 'Introduction: Successful Aging as a Twenty-First-Century Obsession'. In *Successful Aging as a Contemporary Obsession*, edited by Sarah Lamb, 1–23. New Brunswick, NJ: Rutgers University Press.

Lambek, Michael. 2000a. 'The Anthropology of Religion and the Quarrel between Poetry and Philosophy'. *Current Anthropology* 41 (3): 309–20.

Lambek, Michael. 2000b. 'Nuriaty, the Saint and the Sultan: Virtuous Subject and Subjective Virtuoso of the Post-modern Colony'. *Anthropology Today* 16: 7–12.

Lambek, Michael. 2008a. 'Measuring—or Practising Well-Being?' In *Culture and Well-Being: Anthropological Approaches to Freedom and Political Ethics*, edited by Alberto Corsín Jimenez, 115–33. London: Pluto.

Lambek, M. 2008b. 'Value and Virtue'. *Anthropological Theory* 8 (2): 133–57.

Lambek, Michael. 2010. 'Introduction'. In *Ordinary Ethics: Anthropology, Language, and Action*, edited by M. Lambek, 1–36. New York: Fordham University Press.

Lambek, Michael. 2015. *The Ethical Condition: Essays on Action, Person, and Value*. Chicago: University of Chicago Press.

Lambek, Michael. 2016. 'Comment' [on Robbins 2016]. *JRAI* 22 (4): 781–85.

Lambert, Helen. 2005. 'Accounting for EBM: Notions of Evidence in Medicine'. *Social Science and Medicine* 62: 2633–45.

Lasch, Christopher. 1980. *The Culture of Narcissism: American Life in an Age of Diminishing Expectations*. New York: W. W. Norton.

Layard, Richard. 2005. *Happiness: Lessons from a New Science*. London: Penguin Books.

Lee, Andy. 2019. 'A Review of McMindfulness'. *Mindful: Healthy Mind, Healthy Life*, 15 August, https://www.mindful.org/a-review-of-mcmindfulness/ (accessed 30 November 2022).

Lefebvre, Henri. 1991 [1958]. *Critique of Everyday Life*, vol 1: *Introduction*, translated by John Moore. London: Verso.

Leibing, Annette and Silke Schicktanz. 2021. 'Introduction: Reflections on the "New Dementia"'. In *Preventing Dementia? Critical Perspectives on a New Paradigm of Preparing for Old Age* edited byAnnette Leibing and Silke Schicktanz, 1–18. New York: Berghahn Books.

Lempert, Michael. 2013. 'No Ordinary Ethics'. *Anthropological Theory* 13 (4): 370–93.

Lewis, Gwyneth. 2002. *Sunbathing in the Rain: A Cheerful Book about Depression*. London: Harper.

Liberatore, Angela and Silvio Funtowicz. 2003. '"Democratising" Expertise, "Expertising" Democracy: What Does This Mean, and Why Bother?'. *Science and Public Policy* 30 (3): 146–50.

Littlewood, Roland. 1980 'Anthropology and Psychiatry: An Alternative Approach'. *British Journal of Medical Psychiatry* 53: 213–25.

Littlewood, Roland and Simon Dein. 1995. 'The Effectiveness of Words: Religion and Healing among the Lubavitch of Stamford Hill'. *Culture, Medicine, and Psychiatry* 19 (3): 339–69.

Littlewood, Roland and Maurice Lipsedge. 1987. 'The Butterfly and the Serpent: Culture, Psychopathology and Biomedicine'. *Culture, Medicine, and Psychiatry* 11 (3): 289–335.

Littlewood, Roland and Maurice Lipsedge. 1997. *Aliens and Alienists: Ethnic Minorities and Psychiatry* (3rd edition). Middlesex: Penguin Books.

Long, Nicholas J. 2013. 'Political Dimensions of Achievement Psychology: Perspectives on Selfhood, Confidence and Policy from a New Indonesian Province'. In *The Social Life of Achievement*, edited by Nicholas J. Long and Henrietta L. Moore, 82–102. New York: Berghahn Books.

Lopez Donald S., Jr. 2016. 'The Life of the Lotus Sutra'. *Tricycle: The Buddhist Review*, Winter (vol. 27, no. 2). Available at https://tricycle.org/magazine/lotus-sutra-history/ (accessed 30 November 2022).

Low, Carissa. A., Annette. L. Stanton and Julienne E. Bower. 2008. 'Effects of Acceptance-Oriented versus Evaluative Emotional Processing on Heart Rate Recovery and Habituation'. *Emotion* 8: 419–24.

Löwy, Michael and Robert Sayre. 2001. *Romanticism against the Tide of Modernity*, translated by Catherine Porter. Durham, NC: Duke University Press.

LSE. 2006. = London School of Economics and Political Science. Centre for Economic Performance. Mental Health Policy Group (2006). *The Depression Report: A New Deal for Depression and Anxiety Disorders*. London: LSE Research Online. Available at http://eprints.lse.ac.uk/archive/00000818 (accessed 30 November 2022).

Lucas, Marsha. 2013. *Rewire Your Brain for Love: Creating Vibrant Relationships Using the Science of Mindfulness*. Carlsbad, CA: Hay House.

Luhrmann, Tanya M. 2007. 'Social Defeat and the Culture of Chronicity; or, Why Schizophrenia Does So Well Over There and So Badly Here'. *Culture, Medicine, and Psychiatry* 31, 135–72.

Luhrmann, Tanya M. 2012. *When God Talks Back: Understanding the American Evangelical Relationship with God.* New York: Knopf.

Luhrmann, Tanya and Jocelyn Marrow (eds). 2016. *Our Most Troubling Madness: Schizophrenia across Cultures.* Los Angeles: University of California Press.

Lukianoff, Greg and Jonathan Haidt. 2018. *The Coddling of the American Mind: How Good Intentions and Bad Ideas Are Setting Up a Generation for Failure.* New York: Penguin.

Lupton, Deborah. 1997. 'Foucault and the Medicalisation Critique'. In *Foucault, Health and Medicine,* edited by Alan Petersen and Robin Bunton, 94–110. London: Routledge.

Lutz, Catherine. 1985. 'Depression and Translation'. In *Culture and Depression: Studies in the Anthropology and Cross-cultural Psychiatry of Affect and Disorder,* edited by Arthur Kleinman and Byron J. Good, 63–100. Berkeley, CA: University of California Press.

Ma, S. Helen and John D. Teasdale. 2004. 'Mindfulness-Based Cognitive Therapy for Depression: Replication and Exploration of Differential Relapse Prevention Effects'. *Journal of Consulting and Clinical Psychology* 72 (1): 31–40.

Maasen, Sabine and Oliver Lieven. 2006. 'Transdiciplinarity: A New Mode of Governing Science?' *Science and Public Policy* 33 (6): 399–410.

Macaro, Antonia and Julian Baggini. 2015. 'Business on the Mindfulness Bandwagon'. *Financial Times,* 13 March. Available (subscription only) at https://www.ft.com/content/ee65c5e4-c82f-11e4-8fe2-00144feab7de (accessed 30 November 2022).

Mair, Jonathan. 2013. 'Cultures of Belief'. *Anthropological Theory,* 12: 448–66.

Mair, Jonathan. 2018. 'Metacognitive Variety, from Inner Mongolian Buddhism to Post-Truth'. In *Metacognitive Diversity: An Interdisciplinary Approach,* edited by by Joëlle Proust and Martin Fortier, 395–414. Oxford: Oxford University Press.

Manderson, Lenore and Carolyn Smith-Morris (eds). 2010. *Chronic Conditions, Fluid States: Chronicity and the Anthropology of Illness.* New Brunswick, NJ: Rutgers University Press.

Mantos, Manuel, Carolina Segura, Mauricio Eraso, Jean Oggins and Katie McGovern. 2014. 'Association of Brief Mindfulness Training with Reductions in Perceived Stress and Distress in Colombian Health Care Professionals'. *International Journal of Stress Management* 21: 207–55.

MAPPG. 2015a. *Mindful Nation UK: Report by the Mindfulness All-Party Parliamentary Group (MAPPG).* Available at https://www.themindfulnessinitiative.org/mindful-nation-report (accessed 30 November 2022).

MAPPG. 2015b. *Mindful Nation UK: Interim Report of the Mindfulness All-Party Parliamentary Group (MAPPG).* Available at https://issuu.com/omnipsiconsulting/docs/mindful-nation-uk-interim-report-of (accessed 30 November 2022).

Marks, Nic, and Hetan Shah. 2005. 'A Well-Being Manifesto for a Flourishing Society'. In *The Science of Well-Being,* edited by Felicia A. Huppert, Nick Baylis and Barry Keverne, 503–31. Oxford: Oxford University Press.

Marsella, Anthony J. 1978. 'Thoughts on Cross-cultural Studies on the Epidemiology of Depression'. *Culture, Medicine and Psychiatry* 2: 343–57.

Marsella, Anthony J. 1985. 'Culture, Self, and Mental Disorder'. In *Culture and Self: Asian and western perspectives,* edited by Anthony J. Marsella, George A. DeVos and Francis L. K. Hsu, 281–308. London: Tavistock Press.

Martin, Emily. 2010. 'Self-Making and the Brain'. *Subjectivity* 3 (4): 366–81.

Martin, Mike 2006 *From Morality to Mental Health: Virtue and Vice in a Therapeutic Culture.* Oxford: Oxford University Press.

Massie, Graeme. 2021. '"Cry Closet": Amazon Mocked for Creating "AmaZen" Mental Health Box for Warehouse Workers'. *The Independent*, 27 May. Available at https://www.independent .co.uk/news/world/americas/amazon-mental-health-box-workers-b1855386.html (accessed 30 November 2022).

Masuzawa, Tomoko. 2005. *The Invention of World Religions; or, How European Universalism Was Preserved in the Language of Pluralism.* Chicago: University of Chicago Press.

Mattingly, Cheryl. 2014a. 'Moral Deliberation and the Agentive Self in Laidlaw's Ethics'. *HAU: Journal of Ethnographic Theory* 4 (1): 473–86.

Mattingly, Cheryl. 2014b. *Moral Laboratories: Family Peril and the Struggle for a Good Life.* Oakland, CA: University of California Press.

Mattingly, Cheryl. 2017. 'Autism and the Ethics of Care: A Phenomenological Investigation into the Contagion of Nothing'. *ETHOS* 45 (2): 250–70.

Matza, Tomas. 2018. *Shock Therapy: Psychology, Precarity, and Well-Being in Postsocialist Russia.* Durham, NC: Duke University Press.

Mautner, Ori. 2020. 'Cultivation and Conflict: Buddhist-Derived Meditation and Ethical Complexity among Israeli Jews'. Doctoral thesis, University of Cambridge.

McCane-Katz, Elinore F. 2019. *The National Survey on Drug Use and Health: 2019.* Substance Abuse and Mental Health Services Administration (SAMHSA)

McCracken, Lance. M. and Su-Yin Yang. 2008. 'A Contextual Cognitive-Behavioural Analysis of Rehabilitation Workers' Health and Well-Being: Influences of Acceptance, Mindfulness and Value-based Action'. *Rehabilitation Psychology* 53: 479–85.

McCrone, Paul, Sujith Dhanasiri, Anita Patel, Martin Knapp and Simon Lawton-Smith. 2008. *Paying the Price: The Cost of Mental Health Care in England to 2026.* London: King's Fund. Available at https://www.kingsfund.org.uk/sites/files/kf/Paying-the-Price-the-cost-of -mental-health-care-England-2026-McCrone-Dhanasiri-Patel-Knapp-Lawton-Smith-Kings -Fund-May-2008_0.pdf (accessed 30 November 2022).

McDaniel, Justin. 2011. *The Lovelorn Ghost and the Magical Monk: Practicing Buddhism in Modern Thailand.* New York: Columbia University Press.

McDonagh, Melanie. 2014. 'Mindfulness Is Something Worse than Just a Smug Middle-Class Trend'. *The Spectator*, 1 November.

McDonagh, Melanie. 2015 'Don't Chill Out—It Won't Do You or Society Any Good'. *Evening Standard*, 6 May. Available at https://www.standard.co.uk/comment/comment/melanie -mcdonough-don-t-chill-out-it-won't-do-you-or-society-any-good-10275757.html (accessed 30 November 2022).

McGreevey, Sue. 2011. 'Eight Weeks to a Better Brain'. *The Harvard Gazette*, 21 January. Available at https://news.harvard.edu/gazette/story/2011/01/eight-weeks-to-a-better-brain/ (accessed 30 November 2022).

McKay, Francis. 2019. 'Equanimity: The Somatization of a Moral Sentiment from the Eighteenth to the Late Twentieth Century'. *Journal of the History of the Behavioural Sciences*: 1–18.

McKinney, Kelly A. and Brian G. Greenfield. 2010. 'Self-Compliance at "Prozac Campus"'. *Anthropology and Medicine* 17 (2): 173–85.

McMahan, David L. 2004. 'Modernity and the Early Discourse of Scientific Buddhism'. *Journal of the American Academy of Religion* 72 (4): 897–933.

McMahan, David L. 2008. *The Making of Buddhist Modernism*. Oxford: Oxford University Press.

McMahan, David L. and Erik Braun, eds. 2017. *Meditation, Buddhism, and Science*. Oxford: Oxford University Press.

McManus, Sally, Paul Bebbington, Rachel Jenkins and Terry Brugha. 2014. 'Executive Summary'. In *Mental Health and Wellbeing in England: Adult Psychiatric Morbidity Survey 2014*. Leeds: NHS Digital. Available at https://digital.nhs.uk/data-and-information/publications /statistical/adult-psychiatric-morbidity-survey/adult-psychiatric-morbidity-survey-survey -of-mental-health-and-wellbeing-england-2014 (accessed 30 November 2022).

Mehta, Nisha, Orla Murphy and Charlotte Lillford-Wildman (eds). 2014. *Annual Report of the Chief Medical Officer 2013: Public Mental Health Priorities: Investing in the Evidence*. London: Department of Health. Available (online only) at https://assets.publishing.service.gov.uk /government/uploads/system/uploads/attachment_data/file/413196/CMO_web_doc .pdf (accessed 30 November 2022).

Merrit, Maria W., John M. Doris and Gilbert Harman. 2010. 'Character'. In *The Moral Psychology Handbook*, edited by John M. Doris and The Moral Psychology Research Group, 355–401. Oxford: Oxford University Press.

MHF. 2022. 'About Mental Health', https://www.mentalhealth.org.uk/explore-mental-health /about-mental-health (accessed 30 November 2022).

Michaelson, Jay. 2014. 'What if Meditation Isn't Good for You?'. *Daily Beast*, 1 November, updated 14 April 2017, https://www.thedailybeast.com/what-if-meditation-isnt-good-for-you (accessed 30 November 2022).

Mikulas, W. L. 2011. 'Mindfulness: Significant Common Confusions'. *Mindfulness* 2: 1–7.

Miller, Daniel. 2005. 'What Is Best "Value"? Bureaucracy, Virtualism and Local Governance'. In *The Values of Bureaucracy*, edited by Paul du Gay, 233–54. Oxford: Oxford University Press.

Mind 2017 'Mental Health is Everyone's Business: Insurance Charities; Lunchtime Briefings'. https://www.localinstitutes.cii.co.uk/media/9025/birmingham-mind-21-june-2017.pdf (accessed 30 November 2022).

Error! Hyperlink reference not valid. Ministry of Justice. 2013. *Gender Differences in Substance Misuse and Mental Health amongst Prisoners*. London: Ministry of Justice.

Mittermaier, Amira. 2011. *Dreams That Matter: Egyptian Landscapes of the Imagination*. Berkeley, CA: University of California Press.

Moffitt, Terrie E., Louise Arseneault, Daniel Belsky, Nigel Dickson, Robert J. Hancox, HonaLee Harrington, Renate Houts, Richie Poulton, Brent W. Roberts, Stephen Ross, Malcolm R. Sears, W. Murray Thomson and Avshalom Caspi. 2011. 'A Gradient of Childhood Self-Control Predicts Health, Wealth, and Public Safety'. *Proceedings of the National Academy of Sciences* 108 (7): 2693–98.

Moloney, Paul. 2016. 'Mindfulness: The Bottled Water of the Therapy Industry'. In *Handbook of Mindfulness: Culture, Context, and Social Engagement*, edited by Ronald E. Purser, David Forbes and Adam Burke, 269–92. Basel: Springer.

Moody, Oliver. 2015. 'Mindfulness, It Can Mess with Your Head' *The Times*, 22 May. Available at https://www.thetimes.co.uk/article/mindfulness-it-can-mess-with-your-head -7vsmblp93pj (accessed 30 November 2022).

Moyer, Christopher. A., Michael P. W. Donnelly, Jane C. Anderson, Kally C. Valek, Sarah J. Huckaby, Derek A. Widerholt, Rachel L. Doty, Aaron S. Rehlinger, and Brianna L. Rice. 2011. 'Frontal Electroencephalographic Asymmetry Associated with Positive Emotion is Produced by Very Brief Meditation Training'. *Psychological Science* 22: 1277–79.

Mrazak, Michael D., Michael S. Franklin, Dawa Tarchin Phillips, Benjamin Baird and Jonathan W. Schooler. 2013. 'Mindfulness Training Improves Working Memory Capacity and GRE Performance While Reducing Mind Wandering'. *Psychological Science* 24 (5): 776–81.

Myers, Neely, Sara Lewis and Mary Ann Dutton 2015 'Open Mind, Open Heart: An Anthropological Study of the Therapeutics of Meditation Practice in the US'. *Culture, Medicine, and Psychiatry* 39 (3): 487–504.

Nathoo, Ayesha. 2019. 'Relaxation and Meditation'. In *The Oxford Handbook of Meditation*, edited by Miguel Farias, David Brazier and Mansur Lalljee, ch. 15. https://www.oxfordhandbooks.com/view/10.1093/oxfordhb/9780198808640.001.0001/oxfordhb-9780198808640 (accessed 30 November 2022).

Ng, Edwin. 2016. 'The Critique of Mindfulness and the Mindfulness of Critique: Paying Attention to the Politics of Our Selves with Foucault's Analytic of Governmentality'. In *Handbook of Mindfulness: Culture, Context, and Social Engagement*, edited by Ronald E. Purser, David Forbes and Adam Burke, 135–52. Basel: Springer.

Nhat Hanh. 2008. *The Miracle of Mindfulness*. Boston, MA: Rider.

NHS Digital. 2018. *Mental Health of Children and Young People in England, 2017: Summary of Key Findings*. Available at https://digital.nhs.uk/data-and-information/publications/statistical/mental-health-of-children-and-young-people-in-england/2017/2017 (accessed 30 November 2022).

NICE [National Institute for Health and Care Excellence]. 2009. *Depression in Adults* (NICE guideline CG90). London: NICE.

Nolan, James. 2015. 'When It Came to My Depression, Medicine Was More Effective than Mindfulness'. *Vice*, 22 April, https://www.vice.com/sv/article/gqmx44/depression-medicine-mindfulness-304 (accessed 30 November 2022).

Nolan, James L., Jr. 1998. *The Therapeutic State: Justifying Government at Century's End*. New York: New York University Press.

Nolen-Hoeksema, Susan and Jannay Morrow. 1991. 'A Prospective Study of Depression and Posttraumatic Stress Symptoms after a Natural Disaster: The 1989 Loma Prieta Earthquake'. *Journal of Personality and Social Psychology* 61: 115–21.

North, Anna. 2014. 'The Mindfulness Backlash'. *The New York Times*, 30 June. Available at https://op-talk.blogs.nytimes.com/2014/06/30/the-mindfulness-backlash/?_php=true&_type=blogs&_r=0 (accessed 30 November 2022).

North, Maurice. 1972. *The Secular Priests: Psychotherapists in Contemporary Society*. London: Allen & Unwin.

Norton, Philip. 2008. 'Making Sense of Opposition'. *The Journal of Legislative Studies* 14 (1–2): 236–50.

Novas, Carlos and Nikolas Rose. 2000. 'Genetic Risk and the Birth of the Somatic Individual'. *Economy and Society* 29: 485–513.

Nowotny, Helga. 2003. 'Dilemma of Expertise: Democratising Expertise and Socially Robust Knowledge'. *Science and Public Policy* 30 (3): 151–56.

Nuffield Foundation. 2013. *Social Trends and Mental Health: Introducing the Main Findings*. London: Nuffield Foundation.

Nussbaum, Martha and Amartya Sen (eds). 1993. *The Quality of Life*. Oxford: Clarendon Press.

Nyanaponika Thera. 1962. *The Heart of Buddhist Meditation: A Handbook of Mental Training Based on the Buddha's Way of Mindfulness*. London: Rider.

Offer, Avner (ed). 1996. *In Pursuit of the Quality of Life*. Oxford: Oxford University Press.

O'Connor, Anahad. 2015. 'Meditation for a Good Night's Sleep'. *The New York Times*, 23 February. Available at https://well.blogs.nytimes.com/2015/02/23/meditation-for-a-good-nights-sleep/ (accessed 30 November 2022).

Oldmeadow, Harry. 2004. *Journeys East: 20th Century Western Encounters with Eastern Religious Traditions*. Bloomington, IN: World Wisdom.

O'Nell, Teresa. 1998. *Disciplined Hearts: History, Identity, and Depression in an American Indian Community*. Berkeley, CA: University of California Press.

Owen, Alex. 2004. *The Place of Enchantment: British Occultism and the Culture of the Modern*. Chicago: University of Chicago Press.

Pagis, Michal. 2009. 'Embodied Self-Reflexivity'. *Social Psychological Quarterly* 72 (3): 265–83.

Pagis, Michal. 2010. 'Producing Intersubjectivity in Silence: An Ethnographic Study of Meditation Practice. *Ethnography* 11 (2): 309–28.

Pagis, Michal. 2019. *Inward: Vipassana Meditation and the Embodiment of the Self*. Chicago: University of Chicago Press.

Parkin, David. 1985. *The Anthropology of Evil*. Oxford: Blackwell.

Payne, Richard K. 2016. 'Mindfulness and the Moral Imperative for the Self to Improve the Self'. In *Handbook of Mindfulness: Culture, Context, and Social Engagement*, edited by Ronald E. Purser, David Forbes and Adam Burke, 121–34. Basel: Springer.

Peabody, Elizabeth Palmer. 1844. 'The Preaching of Buddha'. *The Dial*, January (vol. 4, no. 3): 391.

Pedersen, Morten A., Kristoffer Albris and Nick Seaver. 2021. 'The Political Economy of Attention'. *Annual Review of Anthropology* 50: 309–25.

Petryna, Adriana. 2002. *Life Exposed: Biological Citizens after Chernobyl*. Princeton, NJ: Princeton University Press.

Pickert, Kate. 2014. 'The Mindful Revolution'. *Time Magazine*, 3 February. Available at http://content.time.com/time/subscriber/article/0,33009,2163560,00.html (accessed 30 November 2022).

Pidgeon, Aileen M., Lucas Ford, and Frances Klaassen. 2014. 'Evaluating the Effectiveness of Enhancing Resilience in Human Service Professionals Using a Retreat-Based Mindfulness with Metta Training Program: A Randomized Control Trial'. *Psychology, Health, and Medicine* 19: 355–64.

Piet, Jacob and Esben Hougaard. 2011. 'The Effect of Mindfulness-Based Cognitive Therapy for Prevention of Relapse in Recurrent Major Depressive Disorder: A Systematic Review and Meta-analysis'. *Clinical Psychology Review* 31: 1032–40.

Plank, Katarina. 2010. 'Mindful Medicine: The Growing Trend of Mindfulness-Based Therapies in the Swedish Health Care System'. *Finnish Journal of Ethnicity and Migration* 5 (2): 47–55.

Plath, Sylvia. 1966. *The Bell Jar*. London: Faber and Faber.

Pollock, Laurence. 2009 'Fit for Purpose'. *The Guardian*, 18 February. Available at https://www.theguardian.com/society/2009/feb/18/mental-health3 (accessed 30 November 2022).

Poulter, Daniel, Nicole Votruba, Ioannis Bakolis, Frances Debell, Jayati Das-Munshi and Gra-
ham Thornicroft. 2019. 'Mental Health of UK Members of Parliament in the House of Commons: A Cross-sectional Survey' [corrected version]. *BMJ Open* 9 (7), https://bmjopen.bmj
.com/content/9/7/e027892corr1 (accessed 30 November 2022).

Prohl, Inken. 2014. 'Buddhism in Contemporary Europe'. In *The Wiley Blackwell Companion to
East and Inner Asian Buddhism*, edited by Mario Poceski, 485–504. Hoboken, NJ: Wiley.

Prothero, Stephen. 1996. *The White Buddhist: The Asian Odyssey of Henry Steel Olcott*. Bloomington: Indiana University Press.

Proust, Joëlle and Martin Fortier (eds). 2018. *Metacognitive Diversity: An Interdisciplinary
Approach*. Oxford: Oxford University Press.

Purser, Ronald. 2015. 'Clearing the Muddled Path of Traditional and Contemporary Mindfulness: A Response to Monteiro, Musten, and Compson'. *Mindfulness* 6 (1), 23–45.

Purser, Ronald. 2019. *McMindfulness: How Mindfulness Became the New Capitalist Spirituality*.
London: Repeater Books.

Purser, Ronald E., David Forbes and Adam Burke (eds). 2016. *Handbook of Mindfulness: Culture,
Context, and Social Engagement*. Basel: Springer.

Purser, Ronald and David Loy. 2013. 'Beyond McMindfulness'. *Huffpost* (US edition), 1 July,
updated 31 August, https://www.huffpost.com/entry/beyond-mcmindfulness_b_3519289
(accessed 30 November 2022).

Purser, Ronald and Joseph Milillo. 2015. 'Mindfulness Revisited: A Buddhist-based Conceptu-
alization'. *Journal of Management Inquiry* 24 (1): 3–24.

Purser, Ronald and Edwin Ng. 2015. 'Corporate Mindfulness is Bullsh*t: Zen or No Zen, You're
Working Harder and Being Paid Less. Salon'. *Salon*, 27 September, https://www.salon.com
/2015/09/27/corporate_mindfulness_is_bullsht_zen_or_no_zen_youre_working_harder
_and_being_paid_less/ (accessed 30 November 2022).

Putnam, Robert D. 2000. *Bowling Alone: The Collapse and Revival of American Community*. New
York: Simon & Schuster.

Pykett, Jessica, Rachel Howell, Rachel Lilley, Rhys Jones and Mark Whitehead. 2016. 'Govern-
ing Mindfully: Shaping Policy Makers' Emotional Engagements with Behaviour Change'.
In *Emotional States: Sites and Spaces of Affective Governance*, edited by Eleanor Jupp, Jessica
Pykett and Fiona M. Smith, 69–84. New York: Routledge.

Pykett, Jessica, Rhys Jones and Mark Whitehead. 2017. 'Introduction: Psychological Governance and Public Policy'. In *Psychological Governance and Public policy: Governing the
Mind, the Brain and Behaviour*, edited by Jessica Pykett, Rhys Jones and Mark Whitehead,
1–20. Oxford: Routledge.

Rabinow, Paul. 1996. 'Artificiality and Enlightenment: From Sociobiology to Biosociality'. In
Rabinow, *Essays on the Anthropology of Reason*, 81–111. Princeton, NJ.: Princeton University
Press,.

Reardon, Jenny. 2007. 'Democratic Mis-haps: The Problem of Democratization in a Time of
Biopolitics'. *BioSocieties* 2 (2): 239–56.

Reed, Adam. 2017a. 'An Office of Ethics: Meetings, Roles, and Moral Enthusiasm in Animal
Protection'. *JRAI* 23 (S1) (special issue: *Meetings: Ethnographies of Organization Process, Bureaucracy, and Assembly*, edited by Hannah Brown, Adam Reed and Thomas Yarrow),
166–81.

Reed, Adam. 2017b. 'Snared: Ethics and Nature in Animal Protection'. *Ethnos* 82 (1), 68–85.

Reich, Wilhelm. 1970 [1946]. *The Mass Psychology of Fascism*, edited by Mary Higgins and Chester M. Raphael. New York: Farrar, Straus and Giroux.

Reveley, J. 2014. 'School-Based Mindfulness Training and the Economisation of Attention: A Stieglerian View'. *Educational Philosophy and Theory* 47 (8): 1–18.

Rhys Davids, Thomas W. 1881. *Buddhist Suttas*. Oxford: Clarendon Press.

Rhys Davids, Thomas W. 2000 [1877]. *Buddhism: Being a Sketch of the Life and Teachings of Gautama, the Buddha*. New Delhi: Asian Educational Services.

Riles, Annelise. 2006. 'Anthropology, Human Rights, and Legal Knowledge: Culture in the Iron Cage'. *American Anthropologist* 108 (1): 52–65.

Robbins, Joel. 2004. *Becoming Sinners: Christianity and Moral Torment in a Papua New Guinea Society*. Berkeley, CA: University of California Press.

Robbins, Joel. 2016. 'What is the Matter with Transcendence?: On the Place of Religion in the New Anthropology of Ethics'. *JRAI* 22 (4): 767–808.

Rose, Jaqueline. 1999. 'Freud in the Tropics'. *History Workshop Journal* 47: 49–67.

Rose, Nikolas. 1985. *The Psychological Complex: Psychology, Politics and Society in England, 1869–1939*. London: Routledge & Kegan Paul.

Rose, Nikolas. 1990. *Governing the Soul: The Shaping of the Private Self*. New York: Routledge.

Rose, Nikolas 1996a. 'Governing "Advanced" Liberal Democracies'. In *Foucault and Political Reason*, edited by Andrew Barry, Thomas Osborne and Nikolas Rose, 37–64. Chicago: University of Chicago Press.

Rose, Nikolas 1996b. *Inventing Our Selves: Psychology, Power, and Personhood*. Cambridge, MA: Cambridge University Press.

Rose, Nikolas. 2007. 'Governing the Will in a Neurochemical Age'. In *On Willing Selves: Neoliberal Politics and the Challenge of Neuroscience*, edited by Sabine Maasen and Barbara Sutter, 81–99. Basingstoke: Palgrave MacMillan.

Rose, Nikolas. 2010. 'Screen and Intervene: Governing Risky Brains'. *History of the Human Sciences* 23 (1): 79–105.

Rose, Nikolas and Joelle M. Abi-Rached. 2013. *Neuro: The New Brain Sciences and the Management of the Mind*. Princeton, NJ: Princeton University Press.

Rose, Nikolas and Paul Rabinow. 2006. 'Biopower Today'. *Biosocialities* 1 (2): 195–217.

Rosenberg, Charles E. 2015. 'Contested Boundaries: Psychiatry, Disease, and Diagnosis'. *Perspectives in Biology and Medicine* 58 (1): 120–37.

Ryff, Carol D., Gayle Dienberg Love, Marilyn J. Essex and Burton Singer. 1998. 'Resilience in Adulthood and Later Life'. In *Handbook of Aging and Mental Health: An Integrative Approach*, edited by Jacob Lomranz, 69–96. New York: Plenum.

Sangharakshita, Bhikshu. 2008 [1952]. *Anagarika Dharmapala: A Biographical Sketch*. Kandy: Buddhist Publication Society.

Sayeau, Michael. 2013. *Against the Event: The Everyday and the Evolution of Modernist Narrative*. Oxford: Oxford University Press.

Scheper-Hughes, Nancy. 1988. 'The Madness of Hunger: Sickness, Delirium, and Human Needs'. *Culture, Medicine, and Psychiatry* 12: 429–58.

Schicktanz, Silke. 2021. 'If Dementia Prevention Is the Answer, What Was the Question? Observations from the German Alzheimer's Disease Debate'. In *Preventing Dementia? Critical*

Perspectives on a New Paradigm of Preparing for Old Age, edited by Annette Leibing and Silke Schicktanz, 65–91. New York: Berghahn Books.

Schieffelin, Edward L. 1985. 'The Cultural Analysis of Depressive Affect: An Example from New Guinea. In *Culture and Depression: Studies in the Anthropology and Cross-cultural Psychiatry of Affect and Disorder*, edited by, Arthur Kleinman and Byron J. Good, 101–33. Berkeley, CA: University of California Press.

Schmidt, Andreas T. 2016. 'The Ethics and Politics of Mindfulness-Based Interventions'. *Journal of Medical Ethics* 42: 450–54.

Segal, Zindel, Mark G. Williams and John D. Teasdale. 2002. *Mindfulness-Based Cognitive Therapy for Depression*. New York: The Guilford Press.

Segal, Zindel, Mark G. Williams and John D. Teasdale. 2013. *Mindfulness-Based Cognitive Therapy for Depression* (2nd edition). New York: The Guilford Press.

Sen, Amartya K. 1999. *Development as Freedom*. Oxford: Oxford University Press.

Sennett, Richard. 1977. *The Fall of Public Man*. London: Penguin.

Shapiro, Shauna L., Kirk W. Brown and Gina M. Biegel. 2007. 'Teaching Self-Care to Caregivers: Effects of Mindfulness-Based Stress Reduction on the Mental Health of Therapists in Training'. *Training and Education in Professional Psychology* 1 (2): 105–11.

Shapiro, Shauna L., Doug Oman, Carl E. Thoresen, Thomas G. Plante and Tim Flinders. 2008. 'Cultivating Mindfulness: Effects on Well-Being'. *Journal of Clinical Psychology* 64 (7): 840–62.

Shapiro, Shauna. L., Gary E. Schwartz and Ginny Bonner. 1998. 'Effects of Mindfulness-Based Stress Reduction on Medical and Premedical Students'. *Journal of Behavioural Medicine* 21: 581–99.

Sharf, Robert. 2017. 'Is Mindfulness Buddhist? (And Why it Matters)'. In *Meditation, Buddhism, and Science*, edited by David L. McMahan and Erik Braun, 198–211. Oxford: Oxford University Press.

Sheringham, Michael. 2006. *Everyday Life: Theories and Practices from Surrealism to the Present*. Oxford: Oxford University Press.

Sherman, Nancy. 1989. *The Fabric of Character: Aristotle's Theory of Virtue*. Oxford: Clarendon Press.

Shore, Cris and Susan Wright. 2000. 'Coercive Accountability: The Rise of Audit Culture in Higher Education'. In *Audit Cultures*, edited by Marilyn Strathern, 57–89. London: Routledge.

Shove, Elizabeth and Arie Rip. 2000. 'Users and Unicorns: A Discussion of Mythical Beasts in Interactive Science'. *Science and Public Policy*, 27 (3): 175–82.

Siegel, Daniel J. 2007. *The Mindful Brain in Human Development: Reflection and Attunement in the Cultivation of Well-Being*. New York: W. W. Norton.

Siegel, Daniel. J. 2013. *Brainstorm: The Power and Purpose of the Teenage Brain*. New York: Penguin Putnam.

Siegel, Daniel J. 2016. *Mind: A Journey to the Heart of Being Human*. New York: W. W. Norton.

Siegel, Daniel J. 2018. *Aware: The Science and Practice of Presence*. New York: Penguin.

Simons, Ned. 2013. 'MPs Slow the Westminster Treadmill with Weekly "Mindfulness" Meetings'. *Huffpost* (UK edition), 1 November, updated 4 November, https://www.huffingtonpost.co .uk/2013/10/30/chris-ruane-parliament-mindfulness_n_4177609.html (accessed 30 November 2022).

Singh, Nirbhay N., Giulio E. Lancioni, Alan S. W. Winton, Ashvind N. Singh, Angela D. Adkins and Judy Singh. 2008. 'Clinical and Benefit–Cost Outcomes of Teaching a Mindfulness-Based Procedure to Adult Offenders with Intellectual Disabilities'. *Behavior Modification* 3 (5): 622–37.

Singh, Nirbhay N., Giulio E., Lancioni, Alan S. W. Winton, Ashvind N. Singh, Angela D. Adkins and Judy Singh. 2011. 'Can Adult Offenders with Intellectual Disabilities Use Mindfulness-Based Procedures to Control Their Deviant Sexual Arousal?' *Psychology, Crime & Law* 17 (2): 165–79.

Singleton, N., R. Bumpstead, M. O'Brian, A. Lee and H. Meltzer. 2003. 'Psychiatric Morbidity among Adults Living in Private Households'. *International Review of Psychiatry* 15: 65–73.

Snodgrass, Judith. 2009. 'Discourse, Authority, Demand: The Politics of Early English Publications on Buddhism'. *TransBuddhism: Transmission, Translations, and Transformation*, edited by Nalini Bushan, Jay L. Garfield and Adam Zablocki, 21–42. Amhurst, MA: University of Massachusetts Press.

Solomon, Andrew. 2001. *The Noonday Demon: An Atlas of Depression*. London: Vintage Books.

Spence, Ruth, Adam Roberts, Cono Ariti and Martin Bardsley. 2014. *Focus On: Antidepressant Prescribing; Trends in Prescribing of Antidepressants in Primary Care* (QualityWatch report). The Health Foundation and the Nuffield Trust. Available at https://www.nuffieldtrust.org.uk/research/focus-on-antidepressant-prescribing (accessed 30 November 2022).

Spiro, Melford E. 1970. *Buddhism and Society: A Great Tradition and Its Burmese Vicissitudes*. New York: Harper & Row.

Stafford, Charles. 2013. 'Ordinary Ethics in China Today'. In *Ordinary Ethics in China*, edited by Charles Stafford, 3–28. (London School of Economics Monographs in Social Anthropology 79). London: Bloomsbury.

Stanley, Steven. 2012. 'Intimate Distances: William James' Introspection, Buddhist Mindfulness, and Experiential Inquiry'. *New Ideas in Psychology* 30: 201–11.

Stengers, Isabelle. 2000. *The Invention of Modern Science*, translated by Daniel Smith. Minneapolis: University of Minnesota Press.

Strathern, Marilyn. 2005. 'Resistance, Refusal and Global Moralities'. *Australian Feminist Studies* 20 (47): 181–93.

Strathern, Marilyn. 2006. 'Useful Knowledge'. *Proceedings of the British Academy* 139: 73–109.

Strauss, Clara, Kate Cavanagh, Annie Oliver and Danelle Pettman. 2014. 'Mindfulness-Based Interventions for People Diagnosed with a Current Episode of Anxiety or Depressive Disorder: A Meta-analysis of Randomised Controlled Trials'. *PLOS ONE* 9, https://doi.org/10.1371/journal.pone.0096110.

Styron, William. 1990. *Darkness Visible: A Memoir of Madness*. London: Vintage Books.

Szasz, Thomas S. 1961. *The Myth of Mental Illness: Foundations of a Theory of Personal Conduct*. New York: Hoeber-Harper.

Tambiah, Stanley. 1990. *Magic, Science, Religion and the Scope of Rationality*. Cambridge: Cambridge University Press.

Tang, Yi-Yuan., Yinghua Ma, Junhong Wang, Yaxin Fan, Shigang Feng, Qilin Lu, Yingbao Yu, Danni Sui, Mary K. Rothbart, Ming Fan and Michael I. Posner. 2007. 'Short-Term Meditation Training Improves Attention and Self-Regulation'. *PNAS* 104 (43): 17152–56.

Taylor, Charles. 1989. *Sources of the Self: The Making of Modern Identity*. Cambridge: Cambridge University Press.

Taylor, Eugene. 1991. 'William James and the Humanistic Tradition'. *Journal of Humanistic Psychology* 31 (1): 56–74.

Teasdale, John, D. 1983. 'Negative Thinking in Depression: Cause, Effect, or Reciprocal Relationship?'. *Advances in Behaviour Research and Therapy* 5 (1): 3–25.

Teasdale, John D. 2009. 'Buddhist Mindfulness-Based Therapy (Case Study on Anxiety, Depression)'. Paper presented at the International Conference on Buddhism and Clinical Psychology: 'Ancient Wisdom and Modern Knowledge', Mahidol University, 6–7 August.

Teasdale, John D., Jan Scott, Richard G. Moore, Hazel Hayhurst, Marie Pope and Eugene S. Paykel. 2000. 'How Does Cognitive Therapy Prevent Relapse in Residual Depression? Evidence from a Controlled Trial'. *Journal for Consulting and Clinical Psychology* 69 (3): 347–57.

Teasdale, John D., Zindel V. Segal and J. Mark G. Williams. 1995. 'How Does Cognitive Therapy Prevent Relapse and Why Should Attentional Control (Mindfulness) Training Help?'. *Behaviour Research and Therapy* 33: 225–39.

Teasdale, John D., Zindel V. Segal, J.M.G. Williams, V. A. Ridgeway, J. M. Soulsby and M. A. Lau. 2000. 'Prevention of Relapse/Recurrence in Major Depression by Mindfulness-Based Cognitive Therapy'. *Journal of Consulting and Clinical Psychology* 68: 615–23.

Teasdale, John D., Robert Taylor and Sarah J. Fogarty. 1980. 'Effects of Induced Elation-Depression on the Accessibility of Memories of Happy and Unhappy Experiences'. *Behaviour Research and Theory* 18 (4): 339–46.

Teper, Rimma and Michael Inzlicht. 2014. 'Mindful Acceptance Dampens Neuroaffective Reactions to External and Rewarding Performance Feedback'. *Emotion* 14 (1): 105–14.

Thaler, Richard H. and Cass R. Sunstein. 2008. *Nudge: Improving Decisions about Health, Wealth, and Happiness*. New Haven, CT: Yale University Press.

Thomas, Paul. 2014. 'Reaching across the Aisle: Explaining the Rise of All-Party Parliamentary Groups in the United Kingdom'. Paper presented at the Political Studies Association 65th Annual International Conference, Sheffield, UK, 31 March–1 April.

Thomson, Mathew. 2006. *Psychological Subjects: Identity, Culture, and Health in Twentieth-Century Britain*. Oxford: Oxford University Press.

Thoreau, Henry David. 1854. *Walden*. Boston: Ticknor & Fields.

Throop, Jason. 2010. *Suffering and Sentiment: Exploring the Vicissitudes of Experience and Pain in Yap*. Berkeley, CA: University of California Press.

Titmuss, Christopher. 2016. 'The Buddha of Mindfulness. The Politics of Mindfulness'. *Christopher Titmuss Dharma Blog: A Buddhist Perspective*, 1January, https://www.christophertitmussblog .org/?s=The+Buddha+of+mindfulness (accessed 30 November 2022).

Tugade, Michele M. and Barbara L. Frederickson. 2004. 'Resilient Individuals Use Positive Emotions to Bounce Back from Negative Emotional Experiences'. *Journal of Personality and Social Psychology* 86: 320–33.

University of Miami. 2014. 'Mindfulness Helps Undergraduates Stay on Track'. *ScienceDaily*, 14 January, https://www.sciencedaily.com/releases/2014/01/140114103042.htm (accessed 30 November 2022).

Van Dam, Nicholas, Marieke Van Vugt, David R. Vago, Laura Schmalzl, Clifford Saron, Andrew Olendzki, Ted Meissner, Sara W. Lazar, Jolie Gorchov, Kieran C. R. Fox, Brent A. Field, Willoughby B. Britton, Julie A. Brefczynski-Lewis and David E. Meyer. 2018. 'Reiterated Concerns and Further Challenges for Mindfulness and Meditation Research: A Reply to Davidson and Dahl'. *Perspectives on Psychological Science* 13: 66–69.

Van Esterik, John L. 1977. 'Cultural Interpretation of Canonical Paradox: Lay Meditation in a Central Thai Village'. Doctoral dissertation, University of Illinois.

Varela, Francisco J. 1999. *Ethical Know-How: Action, Wisdom, and Cognition.* Stanford, CA: Stanford University Press.

Versluis, Arthur. 2001. *The Esoteric Origins of the American Renaissance.* New York: Oxford University Press.

Vogel, Else. 2017. 'Hungers that Need Feeding: On the Normativity of Mindful Nourishment'. *Anthropology and Medicine* 24 (2): 159–73.

Wallace, B. Alan. 2007. *Contemplative Science: Where Buddhism and Neuroscience Converge.* New York: Columbia University Press.

Walsh, Zack. 2016. 'A Meta-critique of Mindfulness Critiques: From McMindfulness to Critical Mindfulness'. In *Handbook of Mindfulness: Culture, Context, and Social Engagement,* edited by Ronald E. Purser, David Forbes and Adam Burke, 153–66. Basel: Springer.

Watters, Ethan. 2010. *Crazy Like US: The Globalization of the American Psyche.* New York: The Free Press.

Wells, Kenneth B., Roland Sturm, Cathy D. Sherbourne and Lisa S. Meredith. 1996. *Caring for Depression.* Boston, MA: Harvard University Press.

Wheater, Kitty. 2017. 'Once More to the Body: An Ethnography of Mindfulness Practitioners in the United Kingdom'. Doctoral thesis, University of Oxford.

White, Geoffrey and Anthony Marsella. 1982. 'Introduction: Cultural Conceptions in Mental Health Research and Practice'. In *Cultural Conceptions of Mental Health and Therapy,* edited by Anthony J. Marsella and Geoffrey M. White, 3–38. Dordrecht: Reidel.

Whitehead, Mark, Rhys Jones, Rachel Lilley, Jessica Pykett and Rachel Howell. 2017. *Neuroliberalism: Behavioural Government in the Twenty-First Century.* London: Routledge.

Wikholm, Catherine. 2015a. 'Seven Common Myths about Meditation'. *The Guardian,* 22 May. Available at https://www.theguardian.com/commentisfree/2015/may/22/seven-myths -about-meditation (accessed 30 November 2022).

Wikholm, Catherine. 2015b. '*Sky News*: Should Buddhism Be on the NHS?'. Twitter,16 May.

Wikholm, Catherine and Miguel Farias. 2015. 'Ommm . . . Aargh'. *The New Scientist,* May [226 (3021)], 28–29. Available at https://www.researchgate.net/publication/276414075_Ommm _Aargh/link/5e8714b9a6fdcca789ed3e22/download (accessed 30 November 2022).

Wilkinson, Iain and Arthur Kleinman. 2016. *A Passion for Society: How We Think about Suffering.* Berkeley, CA: University of California Press.

Wilkinson, Richard and Kate Pickett. 2009. *The Spirit Level: Why Equality is Better for Everyone.* London: Penguin Books.

Williams, Mark and Danny Penman. 2011. *Mindfulness: A Practical Guide to Finding Peace in a Frantic World.* London: Piatkus.

Williams, D.D.R. and Jane Garner. 2002. 'The Case against the "Evidence"'. *British Journal of Psychiatry* 180: 8–12.

WHO. 2012. *Risk to Mental Health: An Overview of Vulnerabilities and Risk Factors*. Available at https://www.who.int/publications/m/item/risks-to-mental-health (accessed 30 November 2022).

WHO. 2020. 'Depression'. https://www.who.int/news-room/fact-sheets/detail/depression (accessed 30 November 2022).

Williams, J. Mark G. and Jon Kabat-Zinn. 2011. 'Introduction: Mindfulness; Diverse Perspectives on Its Meaning, Origins, and Multiple Applications at the Intersection of Science and Dharma'. *Contemporary Buddhism* 12 (1): 1–18.

Wilson, Jeff. 2014. *Mindful America: The Mutual Transformation of Buddhist Meditation and American Culture*. Oxford: Oxford University Press.

Wilson, Jeff. 2017. '"Mindfulness Makes You a Way Better Lover": Mindful Sex and the Adaptation of Buddhism to New Cultural Desires'. In *Meditation, Buddhism, and Science*, edited by David L. McMahan and Erik Braun, 152–72. Oxford: Oxford University Press.

Wolpert, Lewis. 1999. *Malignant Sadness: The Anatomy of Depression*. New York: The Free Press.

Woolf, Virginia. 1925. *Mrs Dalloway*. London: Hogarth Press.

Woolf, Virginia. 1985. 'A Sketch of the Past'. In *Moments of Being* (2nd edition), edited by Jeanne Schulkind, 61–160. Orlando, FL: Harcourt Brace.

Wu, Tim. 2017. *The Attention Merchants: The Epic Struggle to Get Inside Our Heads*. London: Atlantic Books.

Young, Allen. 1995. *The Harmony of Illusions: Inventing Post-Traumatic Stress Disorder*. Princeton, NJ: Princeton University Press.

Zeidan, Fadel, Susan K. Johnson, Bruce J. Diamond and Paula Goolkasian. 2013. 'Mindfulness Meditation Improves Cognition: Evidence of Brief Mental Training'. *Consciousness and Cognition* 19 (2): 597–605.

Zola, Irving K. 1972. 'Medicine as an Institution of Social Control'. *Sociological Review* 20 (4): 487–504.

Zoogman, Sarah, Simon B. Goldberg, William T. Hoyt and Lisa Miller. 2015. 'Mindfulness Interventions with Youth: A Meta-analysis'. *Mindfulness* 6: 290–302.

INDEX

Note: Page numbers in italic type indicate illustrations.

A NOTE ON THE TYPE

This book has been composed in Arno, an Old-style serif typeface in the classic Venetian tradition, designed by Robert Slimbach at Adobe.